"*Raising Body Positive Teens* is a wonderful resource for parents who want to help their kids develop habits that will lead to true, enduring health...replacing the harmful and misleading size-focused 'health' that diet culture offers. The expert team of authors offer countless practical ways to develop a friendship with food and body while honoring culinary traditions from around the world. This book breaks down common misconceptions and replaces them with thoughtful, scientifically sound, weight neutral, and body positive lessons that can be deployed that same day."

—*Jennifer L. Gaudiani, MD, CEDS-S, FAED, Founder and Medical Director of the Gaudiani Clinic and author of* Sick Enough: A Guide to the Medical Complications of Eating Disorders

"This smart, well-researched book guides parents through every hard conversation and stumbling block we're likely to encounter as we work to empower our kids to love and care for their bodies, and to understand the harm caused by anti-fat bias. I'm so grateful to have this on my bookshelf!"

—*Virginia Sole-Smith, author of* The Eating Instinct

"My margin notes had margin notes! I eagerly absorbed the sound wisdom and concrete suggestions in this book, and will be suggesting it to friends, colleagues, and fellow parents for years to come. *Raising Body Positive Teens* is smart, readable, and endlessly helpful."

—*Sara Gilliam, co-author of* Reviving Ophelia: 25th Anniversary Edition

"*Raising Body Positive Teens* provides parents with practical advice, interactive activities, and real-life examples as they support their children through adolescence. The authors are respected experts with extensive experience in mental health, nutrition, and adolescent medicine."

—*Jason Nagata, MD, MSc, Assistant Professor of Pediatrics, University of California*

"How we nurture ourselves and the well-being of our children requires thoughtful awareness. *Raising Body Positive Teens* is the best go-to book for parents on learning how to support, inspire, and navigate teens toward their best possible selves."

—*Dan Tomasulo, PhD, author of* Learned Hopefulness: The Power of Positivity to Overcome Depression *and Academic Director, Spirituality Mind Body Institute Teachers College, Columbia University*

"This is the book we wish our own parents had read when we were teens, and just the balm today's parents are looking for to navigate the messiness of current day diet culture. Perfect for anyone whose own food and body journey has been on the wobbly side of things and wanting something different for our own young people, this gem will be on my go-to recommended list for many years to come."

—*Fiona Sutherland, ADP, RYT. Director, The Mindful Dietitian and Host, The Mindful Dietitian Podcast*

Raising Body
Positive Teens

by the same authors

No Weigh!
A Teen's Guide to Positive Body Image, Food, and Emotional Wisdom
Signe Darpinian, Wendy Sterling, Shelley Aggarwal
Foreword by Connie Sobczak
ISBN 978 1 78592 825 3
eISBN 978 1 78450 946 0

of related interest

The No Worries Guide to Raising Your Anxious Child
A Handbook to Help You and Your Anxious Child Thrive
Karen Lynn Cassiday, PhD
ISBN 978 1 78775 887 2
eISBN 978 1 78775 888 9

The Parents' Guide to Body Dysmorphic Disorder
How to Support Your Child, Teen or Young Adult
Nicole Schnackenberg, Benedetta Monzani and Amita Jassi
Foreword by Rob Wilson and David Veale
ISBN 978 1 78775 113 2
eISBN 978 1 78775 114 9

A Short Introduction to Understanding and Supporting
Children and Young People with Eating Disorders
Lucy Watson and Bryan Lask
ISBN 978 1 84905 627 4
eISBN 978 1 78450 102 0

RAISING BODY POSITIVE TEENS

A Parent's Guide to Diet-Free Living, Exercise, and Body Image

Signe Darpinian, Wendy Sterling, and Shelley Aggarwal

Jessica Kingsley Publishers
London and Philadelphia

First published in Great Britain in 2022 by Jessica Kingsley Publishers
An imprint of Hodder & Stoughton Ltd
An Hachette UK Company

1

Disclaimer: The information contained in this book is not intended to replace the services of trained medical professionals or to be a substitute for medical advice. You are advised to consult a doctor on any matters relating to your health, and in particular on any matters that may require diagnosis or medical attention.

A CIP catalogue record for this title is available from the British Library and the Library of Congress

ISBN 978 1 83997 039 9
eISBN 978 1 83997 040 5

Printed and bound in the United States by Integrated Books International

Jessica Kingsley Publishers' policy is to use papers that are natural, renewable and recyclable products and made from wood grown in sustainable forests. The logging and manufacturing processes are expected to conform to the environmental regulations of the country of origin.

Jessica Kingsley Publishers
Carmelite House,
50 Victoria Embankment,
London, EC4Y 0DZ, UK

www.jkp.com

Contents

Contents

Acknowledgments

We would like to acknowledge those who have assisted us across the lifespan of this project: Anna Lutz, nationally recognized leader and family feeding specialist, for contributing endless hours of her time, her expertise, and her passionate commitment to our diet-free parenting chapter; Riley Nickols, Ph.D., sport psychologist, for sharing his voice and wisdom in our exercise and body image chapters; Dan Tomasulo, Ph.D., author of *Learned Hopefulness: The Power of Positivity to Overcome Depression*, for generously lending his time and techniques for improving body image through micro-goals and hope; Joanna Steinglass, M.D., professor of psychiatry and the associate director of the Center for Eating Disorders at Columbia University Medical Center and the New York State Psychiatric Institute, for her assistance with infusing the habit-based model throughout our exercise chapter; Meeta Singh, M.D., service chief of sleep medicine, and section head and medical director at the Henry Ford Allegiance Sleep Health Center in Michigan, for sharing her expertise and guidance on sleep science; Margaret R. Hunter, certified eating disorder creative arts therapist and author of *Reflections of Body Image in Art Therapy*, for her insights on our social media chapter; Elizabeth Scott, co-founder of The Body Positive, for her insights on expanding the definition of beauty and helping people develop balanced, joyful self-care and a relationship with their bodies that is guided by love, forgiveness, and humor; Kristen Meinzer, culture critic and host of the podcast Movie Therapy with Rafer and Kristen, for offering our readers her brilliant insights into becoming critical viewers of the media through movies; Aaron Flores, registered dietitian nutritionist, for his excerpt on reclaiming the word "fat," and for his life's work helping individuals leave behind the world of diets and body shame; Norman Kim, Ph.D., co-founder of Reasons Eating Disorder Center, for offering their lived experiences of food and culture; Virginia Sole-Smith, author of *The Eating Instinct: Food Culture, Body Image, and Guilt in America*, for fielding questions from parents about diet culture and fatphobia; and Sara Pipher Gilliam, co-author of *Reviving Ophelia: Saving the Selves of Adolescent Girls, 25th Anniversary Edition*, for her expertise on social media wellness, and for her amazing edits that made our words sing.

We are grateful to all of the teens and families we have worked with over the years; thank you for trusting us with your care. We are honored to be part of your journey.

We are endlessly appreciative of our colleagues and mentors, who have been our teachers, friends, and support system across decades of work.

Last but not least, we would like to thank Jessica Kingsley Publishers for believing in us and for their commitment to teen health, diet-free living, and supporting parents in raising body-positive teens.

We would be remiss if we didn't mention those who personally supported and encouraged us from idea to publication.

Signe would like to thank her mother, Sonja Knutsen, who smiled squeamishly when she mentioned a second book project. Sonja quietly and selflessly picked up the pieces to support this single parent in the last stages of book completion. She would also like to thank her daughter, Andie Darpinian, the best thing that has ever happened to her, for her patience through this process, "mostly" not taking it personally, and for not "stabbing our book in the heart," despite that very dramatic threat during a particularly intense writing jag. Signe would also like to thank Holly M. Davies for her ongoing non-judgmental guidance, and always encouraging her to do whatever is her highest and best.

Wendy would like to thank her mentors and colleagues who have helped shape how she thinks about food and weight. She would like to thank her parents, Fran and Stuart Meyer, for their unconditional love and support, and for the gift of raising her in a diet-free household. This gift has offered true peace, happiness, and joy around food, which she, in turn, shares with her daughters and her clients. She thanks daughters Emily and Lexi Sterling for listening to the daily adventures about the writing process, for their amazing creations in the kitchen (which helped sharpen her writing), and for their endless love and laughter. Finally, she would like to thank her husband and partner in parenting, Peter Sterling, for being so patient while she was writing at odd hours, and for his love, friendship, and unwavering support. She is grateful for his true alignment in creating a body-positive household for their family.

Shelley would like to acknowledge her mother and father, Ramey and Vijay Aggarwal; you made me capable. To the beloved family, friends, mentors, and guides who have touched my life, thank you for the grace.

Introductions

SIGNE'S INTRODUCTION

I grew up in the Central Valley region of California, home of the typical Valley Girl. It was the late 1980s and the diet culture era at that time was all about fat-free. I distinctly remember my friends and me discovering fat-free frozen yogurt. We used to eat the you-know-what out of it, because it was marketed as something you could eat without gaining weight. At the time, we weren't paying attention to how the lack of pleasure in our food, due to the absence of fat, left us chasing the satisfaction we weren't getting (when food isn't satisfying it leaves you wanting more). Sugar wasn't yet considered "poison"—that title was reserved for a super cool big hair band (RIP Bret Michaels posters on my walls, #iwontforgetyou).

I remember strutting around with my father's first cellular phone (to be clear, it was in a briefcase and weighed as much as a small dog), desperately hoping it would enhance my status. The only means of communication we had with our peers back then were "live" visits, landline calls, and note passing. And the worst thing that could happen was having your note intercepted by a teacher or a parent (which was humiliating!). I distinctly remember being allowed a 30-minute "talking time" on the phone at night, a stark contrast to the 6–9 hours teens spend on their devices today.

I had briefly heard about bulimia in high school, and I was

vaguely aware of anorexia. Ten years later, after earning my graduate degree in counseling psychology, I knew about the same—nothing. It wasn't until my colleague's daughter almost lost her life to an eating disorder that I embarked on what has become a 20-year journey of endless learning. At that time, my colleague and I both wondered, "How do we know nothing about treating this disorder that is supposedly within our scope of practice? Why wasn't this covered in grad school?"

I have never lost my passion for treating and attempting to prevent eating disorders. I have had the honor of witnessing the recovery process of individuals suffering from eating disorders, and I believe in "recovered." During the COVID-19 pandemic, the demand for eating disorder treatment has outstretched the capacity to address it, which I fear will not resolve for some time. And as you'll see in the chapters to come, as long as our society has fatphobia, we will also have eating disorders. For professionals in the field, the pandemic has sounded the alarm for what we have always known on the front lines of this treatment.

Fast-forward to my daughter, Andie, now 12 years old, for whom I wanted to provide protective factors from the beginning. Andie did a short write-up for my intro and she'd like you to know the following:

> I have grown up always loving my body and showing others that they are beautiful. In my family, with my mom, we will never diet because that's something we would just call weird. You should always love your body whether you are small or tall or fat or skinny. My family is Body Positive. The posters in my room are of empowering women, like the famous singer that I really love named Lizzo. She loves her body very much.

Across the span of my career, I've seen the different body trends sweep our culture, from chiseled abs to thigh gaps to "slim thick." The thing these "ideals" have in common is that they are not typically found in nature. I've seen diet trends move from Weight Watchers and Jenny Craig to more obscure weight-loss fads, all in the name of "health."

I have seen a positive shift in our culture towards awareness. Parents, teachers, caregivers, coaches, and doctors are more able to catch a problem at the first sign (which is the most favorable outcome for treatment), and there are a growing number of healthcare providers using weight-neutral approaches. I truly believe this will be the way of the future. I wrote *Raising Body Positive Teens* in the hope to grow resilience with my daughter and her "friend family," as well as my clients and the culture at large. I hope that it will be a manual that offers both you and your teen tools for strengthening body image and becoming a fearless eater and joyful exerciser.

WENDY'S INTRODUCTION

Last year, my kids came home from school and asked me, "What are pounds? And why would someone want to lose them?" They had overheard two teachers talking about calories, and how they had "gained so much weight over the holidays." I was furious. Did these teachers even know how dangerous this language was, or that dieting is the biggest predictor of eating disorders?

"Diets don't work," I told my girls, my blood boiling. This was the same thing I remember my mother telling me when I was younger. She was adamant, after having a few failed dieting attempts herself, that, quite simply, diets don't work. Decades later, there I was, now passing the same message along to my own children.

Fast-forward to the time when I was waiting for a tennis court with my ten-year-old daughter, and the man in front of us said, "Gee, the courts are so full; everyone is burning off their holiday food." It was right after Thanksgiving, and the ease with which he offered up this statement in front of my child was concerning, and, of course, not surprising. Weight loss, dieting, and compensatory movement are everywhere, at every turn.

Kids hear confusing messages about food starting at an early age, from parents, friends, relatives, teachers, coaches—anyone! Diet messages tell kids that something is wrong with their bodies, increase body shame, and teach them to fear foods. Research shows that these messages put kids at risk for the development of an eating disorder. I have been an adolescent and sports dietitian, with a specialty in eating disorders, for more than 20 years. I have devoted my life's work to fighting back against diet culture and helping teens navigate confusing nutrition messages.

We published *No Weigh!* in 2018, to teach teens how to adopt a non-diet approach to nutrition. Although I turned down the project initially several times—I was writing *How to Nourish Your Child Through an Eating Disorder* at the same time—Signe refused to allow me to say no. (I'm pretty sure her exact words were "No Weigh! You *have* to join us!") Working alongside an adolescent medicine doctor (Shelley) and adolescent therapist (Signe) was a perfect fit, since my work typically utilizes the input and collaboration from a variety of disciplines in treating my patients. Plus, having three authors was excellent for settling writing disputes, especially around Signe's questionably funny 1980s references. If two of us agree, the not-joke-joke gets cut. In *No Weigh!* we taught teens that all bodies are good bodies, and wrote about pubertal development, stress management, sleep, exercise, managing hunger and satiety, why diets don't work, and more.

We were surprised to hear how many parents told us they read *No Weigh!* This indicated there was a real hunger for a book entirely for parents that could help them help their child develop a friendship with food and body. In this book, we include many of the same topics as in *No Weigh!* and also add how to manage social media use, establishing and setting boundaries, diet-free parenting tips, and more. Writing this book has been helpful for me as a parent, and we hope it helps you to create a house that is a place of safety for raising your child and building confident eaters.

SHELLEY'S INTRODUCTION

I was about six, and we were at a family friend's house for dinner. I don't remember anything about the meal but I remember the cake. This was some GOOD cake. I got a piece and absolutely wanted more. So, when the host asked if I was ready for slice two, I'm almost completely certain my "little kid" eyes became cartoon-sized as the thought bubble "YES! Yes, please" appeared above my head. But before I could say anything, my beloved and stern elder family member, who is ten feet tall in this memory, answered for me, with a simple and finite "No, she's had enough." That's pretty standard grown-up stuff trying to regulate a kid. But while these words were simple enough, the moment was so much more than the words.

In addition to the "No, she's had enough," there was a look—that look that every kid knows. It's the one that says, "You better (insert expectation) and don't you dare question me." I don't know if there was a cake emergency—maybe there wasn't enough for everyone—but I know that the look hurt. I remember the feeling of disappointment, some fear, and the force of the unspoken message: you're eating too much. My infant and toddler cuteness had evolved to childhood fatness, and as I grew older, that became less and less acceptable. So, as I grew, I received more and more messages about things like self-control and willpower and weight loss.

I come from a bountiful Indian culture, in which food is at the heart of everything. I recognize that this is true for most, if not all, cultures, but I know the experience of being an

Indian-American person. In my memory, I wasn't fat in India. I wasn't unacceptable there and the term "moti" (loosely translated meaning little fatty, feminine version), a nickname that I still have with some family members, was one of affection and even joy. My mom tells stories all the time about how she used to eat multiple bananas at one go as an adolescent, and how she could eat at any time of the day as a kid. She belly laughs when she talks about her older brother teasing her and asking her if she wanted to eat some sweets. She tells me about sitting straight up and happily eating as he slowly fed her (laughing the whole time!) the delicious dessert he tempted her with. So, what's so funny about this? Well, she was asleep when he asked her and she had enough wherewithal and awareness about wanting sweets to sit up, eat, and fall right back to sleep. My mom loves her food!

My mother's childhood stories don't vilify or stigmatize food. My aunts and uncles of that generation eat with joy, too. They talk about recipes and joke about memories and mention the delicious items that they relished during holidays or special family gatherings. They talk about going to India Gate after dinner for a family outing and surrounding the ice cream vendors, as one by one all the children and then the adults got their ice cream. They mainly talk about when so-and-so said that or so-and-so did that. Food is occasionally the star of the story, but most often it's just one delightful player in the cast of characters of their memories.

I hear different rhetoric from the younger generation, more speaking about needing to lose weight or change their diet. I hear about how they have switched from traditional ghee (clarified butter) to "less fattening" oils. In those instances, I wonder if they (we) are losing our connection, not only to the joy of food but to a kind of ease with living life. It feels to me that my parents' and grandparents' culture was more accepting of diverse body sizes and food wasn't the enemy. I'm not sure exactly when that changed—if it changed for some—but for me, that shift happened when we moved to the West. Being skinny wasn't just another neutral descriptor of a body type. In the Western world, it was a highly valued, aspirational goal mandated for all. Narrow ideas of "good" and "bad" bodies or of "beauty" cut across cultures, and Indian culture is no different. The reality is that these ideas are universal, and I don't know that I would have avoided them growing up in an Eastern culture either. I can only speak to the experience that I did have.

The night of the great cake incident was shortly after we had been to the doctor and my family was told that I was too heavy. My adorable chubby baby body, which had previously been part of my "happy fat kid" identity, suddenly became the reason for medical concern. The same elder that in another context wouldn't have even noticed that I had taken more cake now felt they had to actively stop me from having extra. During the great cake incident, I felt betrayed by the person who I thought saw me as perfect, by the body that I had very little hand in building, and by the favorite dessert that could now, apparently, hurt me. I lost three friendships at that moment.

Every child needs compassionate limits, even with food, at times. It wasn't the "No, she's had enough" that was painful; it was the look. In truth, it was the look in the context of being told that I was fat and that there was something wrong with who I am. My child's mind had no way of differentiating my size from my personhood. So, when a medical professional, someone who I assumed knew "everything," said that there's something wrong with my weight, I understood it as "There's something wrong with Shelley." In my culture, traditionally, you do not question doctors. If a doctor says lose weight, then you lose weight or avoid going back to their office or jump behind something and hope they don't see you if you cross paths in the community. What you don't do—or, at least, what we didn't do when I was a child—is question their authority.

That same lack of questioning has led many to personalize and internalize misguided health messages. I became a doctor to help. At its core, that's the whole of the reason that I chose my profession. Being a physician is not easy, and over the years I've seen the hard work, dedication, and tireless effort of amazing colleagues and friends overlooked and undervalued. I have been mentored and guided by creative, dedicated people who have sacrificed their own health for the sake of others and their profession. I am proud to be part of this extraordinary group of professionals, and I fully acknowledge and respect the commitment of the humans who are physicians and healers. But—you knew this was coming—medicine hasn't done a particularly great job when it comes to education and guidance on nutrition.

I bought into the messages of my medical training when I was told that someone who is heavy is unhealthy. Modern medical training is shifting, but traditionally the standard line has been to recommend weight loss if someone is out of the parameters of acceptable and "normal" weight. Typically, medical education has not considered a broader view, one that looks at an individual's lifestyle, activity level, regulated and joyful eating, personal stressors and how those could be contributing to body and physical health (and psychological health, too), or the host of other variables that are part of our physical experience. My training emphasized that if a patient's body mass index (BMI) was elevated, that was bad, and something had to be done about it. I, and most Western medicine doctors, learned the same spiel about cutting sugary beverages, decreasing fatty and rich foods, and increasing exercise (whether you like it or not), all in an effort to get weight down to a number in the "normal" range. Unfortunately, this spiel not only doesn't help, but in many cases it backfires. Remember the great cake incident?

As you read through this book, know that our trio has worked to unravel the damaging messages of diet culture, in an effort to build or enhance your and your teen's relationship with food and body, so that it is aligned with personal goals, values, and true well-being. In this book, we explore several key topics: teen development and puberty, managing stress and how it relates to mindful eating, sleep, movement for all bodies, diet-free parenting, diet-free meal prep, and parenting in the era of social media, among other topics. This content is designed for parents and caretakers including grandparents, guardians, and all those who have a beloved teen in their lives. We aim to provide relatable information and the opportunity to explore core concepts through interactive explorations.

Realistically, we cannot vaccinate our children against diet culture and faulty messages about "health," but we can help build resilience and model the self-affirming behaviors we want to grow in our homes. As you read this book, reflect on your own experiences, and whether you have a friendship with food. Think about how that has influenced you in your approach to parenting and guiding your teen about food and body. We request that you be compassionate with yourself, as some sections will trigger memories and ideas that may be challenging. Conversely, we hope that this book will prompt problem solving, celebration, and creativity as you consider new approaches to your own friendship with food and body. So, get comfortable, get a pen or pencil, grab some cake (if you like), and let's go...

How to Use This Book

As mentioned, this book is designed to be an interactive resource and toolkit that supports parents and caretakers in understanding and navigating their child's teen years. We offer parents several strategies for helping children to develop peace with their body right from the beginning. The goal is to cultivate a friendship with self which also means a friendship with food. Food is at the heart of many experiences and blended into moments of celebration, mundane family rituals, and even events related to grief and comfort. Food is much more than the ingredients on a menu or the items on a plate. Like a good friendship, a relationship with food should be defined by respect, trust, joy, and a willingness to address one's needs. While the aim of this book is to inform parents in an effort to support their teens, that happens best when a parent or caretaker is supported themselves. So we ask you to look not just at your teen's behaviors, thoughts, and feelings, but also at your own. We have included many reflective explorations throughout the book and we encourage you to do these individually and with your teen as you see fit. The book is structured so that foundational principles such as growth and development, stress, and sleep are towards the beginning, but we encourage you to read the chapters in a way that works for you. So, if you want to go immediately to "Diet-free Parenting," or another section, go for it.

We suggest that you use the remaining space in this chapter to enter any goals that you may have as you read. Come back to it to jot down thoughts, ideas, or questions. Remember this book is meant for you as much as it is for your teen, so use it in a way that works for you.

Chapter 1

You Made It Through Puberty, and Your Teen Will, Too!

The teen years are defined by transitions and filled with change. Most often, these years are linked to images of an awkward youth who is unpredictable, pubertal, and always angry. While this can be true at times, we believe teenagers get a bad rap. Adolescence is one of the most dynamic times in anyone's life. It can be filled with wonder, newness, exploration, some challenges, and also joy. When these years are framed as "difficult," and teens are defined as individuals at the mercy of their hormones, the potential for cooperation and communication between parents and kids can be underestimated and undermined. Most kids get along with their parents, even if they don't always agree with them. (By the way, you don't want your teen to always agree with you. Trust us, you don't...more on that later.) Most kids look to parents and guardians for direction, and often find their own path by repeating modeled behaviors, and also by testing boundaries with those closest to them. When equipped with the right information about the anticipated physical, emotional, and cognitive changes during these wonder years, parents and guardians can function more effectively as guides and mentors to their young person.

Caretakers have more agency now than ever before to inoculate children against toxic cultural messages regarding food and body. Think back to your own teen years—good, bad, or mixed. A lot happened. Your body changed and you became a different person between the time that you entered Teenageville and the time that you left it. You probably gained most of your adult height between ages 10 and 20. Your voice changed. And your ability to think about and discuss more complex topics evolved in ways that allowed you to build towards adult decision making.

Your teen is experiencing all of this and much more right now. Every generation has unique challenges. This modern world allows us to share information in unprecedented ways. The simple click of a button connects us to people around the globe. While many older individuals have adjusted to the realities of 21st-century life, today's teens are growing up with social media, remote learning, online living, climate change, and youth-driven activism as normal in the experience of being human. Online living has transformed the way in which humans experience themselves, each other, and the world. What used to be a trip to the library or a discussion with a trusted friend, family member, or mentor is now a quick Google search. Easy access does not always equate to quality information, and caretakers and teens must learn to be discerning consumers of click-and-go culture.

When parents are empowered with accurate information, particularly about adolescent development, they can gain insight into their teen's needs. This can help with talking to—and, more importantly, understanding—their child. Despite having weathered your own adolescence, it can be agonizing and confusing to watch your beloved and equally befuddled child go through the struggles of "teendom." In some cases, simple conversations can become tense encounters, leading parents to swear that their gentle child has been body-snatched and replaced by a new being. This person looks just like the kid you once knew, but it feels as if your sweet and adoring little one has been secretly replaced with a less-sweet, not-so-adoring, and kinda gangly, acne-prone teen. We say this in some jest, and we encourage you to retain a sense of humor...because you will need it! However, we also understand that some parents and guardians feel helpless in situations related to their teenagers, particularly when arguments arise or disagreements can't be easily resolved. It can be difficult for parents to keep up with the rapid changes of the teen years, especially in light of modern technology. *But it is possible.* Knowledge and insight about development and how it influences physical growth and behavior can help us feel more at ease and hopeful about navigating these years. In this chapter, we offer evidence-based information and discuss what parents can do to help their adolescents when it comes to not only accepting but also celebrating their changing body.

PUBERTY

Puberty is the time in life during which humans—males, females, non-binary, and gender-fluid individuals—go through a growth process in which their body changes from being that of a kid to the body of a young adult. It can be quite "normal" for a biological male to start puberty at age 9. It can also be totally "normal" for this young person's brother or cousin to start the same process at age 14. Thus the range of normal pubertal onset can be between the ages of 9 and 14 years old for a male. The process of completing puberty can take a few years, and the rate at which puberty progresses is also person-specific. That's not to say that most people won't have the same general experiences or move through puberty in about the same amount of time. However, while most people will develop very similarly, they will also have unique experiences because of their own biology, their genetics, and their environment.

Some will follow a different course entirely. The word "normal" is presented in quotes because there is no absolute "normal." There are ranges of human development, and even within these ranges some people fall out of the "normal." Thus, we encourage parents and caretakers not to use age as the predominant marker for interpreting where a young person should be developmentally, how they should behave, or what they should understand. Kids, teens, and young adults can be at different stages of personal development, independent of their peers of the same age. Two biological males who are both 12 years old could be at two starkly different stages of physical development—for example, one who has not yet started puberty and the other who is three years into puberty—and that's okay. Therefore, understanding teen development can help with relating to and also aligning with your adolescent. This allows you to troubleshoot and problem-solve according to their developmental stage. It can help normalize the reality of being human, if there is true agreement that everyone is different and there is no one right way of being, even within puberty. We are all unique and that is the most "normal" thing about us.

Puberty is all about change. It is the time when most humans start growing into their adult bodies and progressing through important milestones. However, physical growth is only one aspect of human development. Humans also experience social and emotional growth, as well as cognitive growth, during the adolescent years. So that concept of "normal" is further expanded when we think of all of these other trajectories. Adolescents and young adults can be at a different point in each of these different areas and maybe even others. They may be biologically earlier to start puberty, but emotionally younger, and yet cognitively advanced. Parents may feel frustrated because their child is not "on track" with a peer or isn't following the developmental trajectory of an older sibling.

Some teens struggle to understand concepts or might move in a way that is clumsy and unlike their agile peers of the same age. Caretakers and teens can fall victim to the inevitable comparisons—"Well, so-and-so is doing great in math," or "Ben's finish time was amazing and you two are training the same amount." The misconception that everyone should be at the same level at the same age is simply inaccurate, and the comparison game hurts everyone.

Generally, biological females will start to develop breasts and then progress to having their periods within a few years. They will experience hair growth in their armpits and genital areas. Biological males will have some of the same changes in reference to hair growth and will also note a deepening voice and the growth of their genitalia. Most adolescents will gain height and have changes in the size and shape of muscles. Kids, especially girls, will notice body adipose (fat) deposition in some parts of the body more than others; this happens differently from the ways males deposit adipose tissue. What does this mean for you and your teen? It means navigating an evolving body shape and size.

If you think back to your own childhood and adolescence, your body at age 10 was physically very different from the one you inhabited by 17, which was again different from your 25-year-old body. This is due to the expected physical and biological changes related to human growth. All humans, boys and girls, will have growth spurts during puberty. Adequate nutrition is fundamental to healthy development and maximizing one's physical potential. Like a plant that requires sunlight, air, soil, and water to grow, bodies need food, vitamins, minerals, fats, carbohydrates, proteins, and many other things to grow.

In addition to a variety of foods, it is vital that teens eat sufficient quantities of food. Eating too little can interrupt growth and development, and impact not only current health but also long-term health outcomes. Adolescents are building the body that they will live in for the rest of their life. While the body is dynamic and can change throughout life, there are key developmental points at this age that may have long-term implications. For example, peak bone mass is generally achieved by late adolescence and young adulthood. An individual may rely on this peak bone density for their lifetime.[1] Someone who has not established a strong foundation may be more at risk for fractures when they are older. Studies also show that teens who diet and engage in caloric restriction are not only at risk for developing eating disorders (which you will hear more about throughout this book) but can also experience adverse effects on their developing bones.[2] Thus, adequate and diverse nutritional intake during this critical growth period is vital for long-term health. One major misunderstanding in our culture is that weight gain is abnormal. Gaining weight is a necessity in the teen years. Just like bones need to grow in length and gain density, other parts of the body, such as muscles, organs, and even the brain, are developing and maturing. Did you know that 60 percent of the brain is adipose (fat) tissue? It's trendy for our culture to promote anti-fat messaging, but actually adipose is critical for the body's basic functions and for human beings to thrive!

Girls and boys distribute adipose tissue in their bodies differently. Girls can have more adipose in their arms and around their thighs, hips, and abdomens. This is one of the reasons that the bodies of boys and girls start to look different as teens go through puberty. Girls develop more rounded hips and waists. However, various cultures have created false values about some body shapes and sizes, stigmatizing bodies that don't fit societal norms of thinness or tallness, and so on. Some people will naturally settle at a higher weight, and others at a lower weight, while still others will hang out somewhere in the middle. This is all normal, and weight in and of itself does not indicate whether anyone is healthy, attractive, or worthy.

It is critical that this message is repeated to all individuals—and especially to children and teens—so that false and detrimental beliefs about weight, body image, and health are not inadvertently imparted at key points of emotional development. We are all influenced by generations of genetic material (genes), as well as our current living environments (food access, activity levels, nutritional culture), and the size and shape of humans are wonderfully variable, even among family members. Think of it this way: if every single member of your family ate exactly the same thing, all of you would still have different body types. Unfortunately, weight has been overvalued as a marker of health. We discourage using weight to determine any aspect of health. Instead, we want caretakers and youth to use body satisfaction, satiety, mindful and enjoyable eating, energizing movement, and personal well-being, defined in deeply personal ways, to be the markers of health.

EXPLORATION: "Grow Your Own Way"

We encourage you to explore ideas of what it means to develop "normally" in modern society.

- ▶ What are some of your beliefs about "normal" adolescent development?

- ▶ Can you recall any messages that you received about your own adolescent body?

- ▶ Can you recall any messages that you received about your eating habits during your teen years?

- ▶ Were these messages positive, negative, or neutral?

- ▶ Were these messages different based on gender?

- ▶ Does your teen's experience seem similar or different to yours?

- ▶ How would you modify any negative messages?

- ▶ How would you like to feel, think, and behave in the future when it comes to food and body?

Ask ALL the Questions

In this chapter, we discussed adolescent development as it is experienced by most people. However, some teens may experience developmental stages that are different from their peers, and in some cases, those experiences may be defined as "abnormal," when considered from a medical framework. Some people may start puberty before age 8 or 9, and others may note that they have not had any signs of pubertal changes even beyond age 14. If you have concerns about how your teen is developing, talk to your doctor and don't hesitate to ask questions. Don't avoid the conversation, as puberty is a natural part of development and it's okay to talk about it. Sometimes progressing through puberty too early or too late can be due to medical reasons, so having the conversation with a medical professional will give you information and offer insight into what's happening, and if additional evaluations are needed.

Chapter 2

Learning Our Stress System

Stress is a part of life. Often, it's not about whether or not we have stress; it's about how we react to it. When we're stressed, the brain becomes over-engaged, making it difficult to see the light at the end of the tunnel. Understanding the stress system is central to eating mindfully in modern society. Food peace starts with inner peace.

In this chapter, we talk broadly about the physiology of stress, to give you an understanding of stress as a concept as well as a lived experience. We hope to give you some comfort, too, that stress is normal and can even be healthy!

We asked some of our favorite teens and tweens to tell us about the most stressful, anxiety-inducing things they've ever experienced or can imagine. They delivered.

- When my mom rolls up to pick me up from school and her windows are down and she's blasting Miley Cyrus and singing along. I am not making this up.

- Getting out of a swimming pool and feeling like everyone is looking at my body.

- Running into all of your friends hanging out together, without you.

- Buying my first bra. My mom asked a saleswoman for help and I wanted the floorboards to just devour me right then.

- When my big sister yelled down the aisle to ask what kind of deodorant I wanted.

- Being late to school and having to walk in with the older kids...so awkward!

- Messing up or losing my place when I'm giving a presentation in class.

- Getting a boner at school and trying to act all chill while you cover it up with your book.

How stress "shows up" can be different for all of us. Many people experience physical symptoms such as headaches, muscle tension, or stomachaches. Some people will tell you that they feel as if their heart is racing or their hands are shaking and sweaty when they are anxious, worried, or angry. Emotions, experiences, and ideas can trigger physical reactions and stress responses. We often link positive emotions with understandable physical reactions (think "butterflies" with excitement or flushed cheeks with romantic feelings or embarrassment). Heightened states of positive emotions are similar to stress responses—although they are associated with more pleasurable feelings, they are a result of similar internal chemistry. The point is that emotions, ideas, and experiences can trigger physical reactions in the body, some of which are visible to others (red cheeks) and some of which are known only to us (a pounding heart).

In this chapter, we discuss some of the pitfalls of repeated or prolonged stress. However, the experience of stress can be very positive. (Yes, really!) For many, deadlines are motivators that lead to finishing chores or projects. A life without challenges wouldn't be very interesting, and the reality is that we need stress and the biological responses associated with it to be able to do complex things. Overcoming difficult situations that challenge us emotionally and physically can be among the most meaningful experiences in many people's lives. These situations often end up being rewarding, or at least becoming key learning points that inform future decision making. In reasonable bursts, and with an appropriate emotional and physical return to baseline well-being, stress adds to life and is beneficial in many ways. However, prolonged, chronic, and overly intense stress is harmful and has physical and emotional consequences.

When it comes to stress, one can broadly think of the parts of the autonomic nervous system (ANS): the sympathetic nervous system (SNS) and the parasympathetic nervous system (PNS). The SNS and PNS exert opposite controls in the body. The SNS operates in protection mode and is linked fundamentally with activity and stress, whereas the PNS is associated less with activity and more with relaxation. The body is never this binary or simple, but it does have clever tools and tricks for survival. Think of your SNS as the body's emergency response system. A call comes in ("Oh no, I have to give a presentation to leadership in ten minutes") and triggers the built-in safety systems in the body. Your SNS activates and sends the fire department (adrenaline) and paramedics (cortisol) and even law enforcement (other biochemical responses) out to protect you. Overall, this is great. You have an efficient, coordinated, and quick crisis management system. But what happens when the trigger ("WHAT? I have to monitor my child's online learning, prep dinner, and have another presentation done tomorrow!") becomes a frequent occurrence? Now, the same protective system is being activated repeatedly. Even if you're not calling emergency services daily, consistently engaging the stress response will lead to a depletion of resources, impacts on health, and fatigue (emotional and cognitive).

The SNS reacts quickly to help deal with a perceived threat. You may have heard of the "fight or flight" response. An example frequently used in biology classes is that of a prehistoric human being chased by a saber-toothed tiger. We consider two choices: stay and fight, or run like hell! Now, let's jump ahead to the 21st century. Our calm minds know the difference between a tiger chasing us and the competing priorities of our overly busy modern lives. However, our stressed minds and our body's emergency response systems may not. A threat is a threat, and your body is looking for a way to survive it. Through a coordinated effort between nerves and hormones, signals are sent out to the body. This leads to reactions that raise blood pressure to get more blood to muscles and vital organs. The heart rate increases to pump more blood, and an increased breathing or respiratory rate brings extra oxygen to the rescue. The brain sends signals to the eyes, and the pupils dilate to let in more light to allow us to see better. Digestion is not a biological priority during an emergent situation, so blood is shunted away from the intestines and reallocated to "high needs" areas, such as muscles to allow for running or fighting. The body dilates some blood vessels to get more blood out. Increased blood flow to the skin and dilation of some blood vessels are visible as blushing.

Here's something that many people don't know: we have yet another nervous system, the enteric nervous system (ENS), that resides in our gastrointestinal (GI) or digestive tract. Scientists have even referred to the GI tract as the second brain. So, for some, and maybe many, stress shows up in their gut. This can be stomach pain. It can be a change in appetite (increase or decrease). It might even be nausea or vomiting, diarrhea or constipation. You've likely known at least one person who said that they threw up before a high-stress moment, such as a performance or presentation. Once again, there is no "right" way to be stressed and different people will have different biological responses and personal experiences. During a high-stress time, some people may avoid food altogether and have no appetite. Others may seek out food—more specifically, certain types of food. People may eat just to sustain themselves and others may eat to comfort themselves. It's hard to eat in response to the body's wisdom when the nervous system is in fight or flight, and the priority is just getting through a stressful situation.

The reality is that stress impacts not only how we digest food but also how we eat it. Certain people may eat on the go without pause and not really taste what they are eating. Others may eat well into the higher ranges of the Hunger Meter (Chapter 6) without paying attention to hunger or satiety cues. Usually, these patterns, which are being driven by stress, do not align with mindful, intentional, and nourishing eating.

Multiple stress hormones can trigger these and many other physical changes within seconds, in order to help a human deal with a moment of crisis or, importantly, what *feels* like a moment of crisis. The body's ability to adapt and adjust to the present moment is extraordinary, and in short, intermittent bursts, the stress response is beneficial as it allows us to meet the moment and deal with the stressor. However, these same internal conditions, when experienced chronically for prolonged periods, can wear on the mind and body. Individuals become at increased risk for hypertension (high blood pressure), inflammation, sleep dysregulation, diabetes, digestive problems, and other health conditions. Also, keep in mind that individuals can have more than just a flight or fight response. Some people, particularly children, may have an immobility response and freeze. This may look like a disconnect, but it is as much about surviving a potential threat as fighting or fleeing. Still others may pass out. There is no exact way to be stressed; everyone's body can react differently. The nervous system is fundamentally a friend but, if overused, it can become a friend that makes life harder and less fun. These principles are universal and apply to all humans, teens and adults. By gaining insight into the stress response for yourself, we are hoping that you will also gain insight into how your teen is experiencing and reacting to their stressors.

We haven't discussed the PNS much, and this is the part of the ANS that you are recruiting through techniques such as deep breathing and mindful observation of your internal and external experiences. Deep, slow, and rhythmic breathing engages the PNS, and through a series of internal hormonal shifts and biochemical signals, the body is instructed to slow down. Heart rate decreases, blood pressure drops, and cortisol levels decrease, to name a few internal changes. The body and brain are distanced from the need to survive a threat and this shift may help with taking a broader view of the situation at hand. Through active redirection and slowed breathing, the panic you're feeling about giving that presentation in ten minutes could change to the realization that you are a content expert, and that's why you have been asked to discuss the topic. Even if you're not the expert, a bit of space between yourself and the high-stress situation will only support you in being able to deal with the circumstances. So, while the racing heart won't entirely go away, the panic may settle and allow for more clarity. Similarly, panic doesn't help digestion. It's better to be relaxed when eating and digesting food. This allows for attunement to one's true needs, enables intentional decision making about what to eat, and supports understanding when you're at a satisfying stopping point. Through awareness, or mindful eating, the goal is to hook into personal subtle cues and understand your own hunger and fullness.

We are best at what we do most often, and recruiting the

relaxation response is a daily practice. In the simplest terms, someone can become great at deep breathing, mindfulness, and robustly recruiting their PNS. Alternatively, unchecked stress that is creating hardship can lead to frequent activation of the SNS. Neither one of these is inherently wrong—they're just biology. However, one set of responses and reactions may lead to more ease and the ability to cope with challenging moments and make nourishing food choices, whereas repeated, difficult-to-manage stress responses will ultimately take a toll. Finally, if someone is experiencing a prolonged sense of worry and/or physical symptoms of chronic stress, there can be medical and mental health reasons for this, including anxiety. That's worth a conversation with a medical or mental health professional.

EXPLORATION: Journaling

Journaling as a tool can be very healing. It can take the worry out of your mind and anchor it to the page. Through this practice, we can process complex feelings, objectively review a difficult situation, or simply commit our feelings to paper. If you prefer writing on paper, do that. If you prefer typing, do that. However, if you're planning this exploration in the late evening or before bed, we would suggest using a pencil/pen and paper to avoid screen time before sleeping.

- ▸ What went well today?

- ▸ What went poorly today?

  - – Do I need to do something to improve this situation?

  - – What can I do to improve the situation? (When feelings of stress are particularly high, it can be helpful to focus on what is possible in the time available.) As you think about this question, start with self-compassion and reasonable expectations.

EXPLORATION: Breathe

Stress doesn't have to be a negative experience. With some perspective and an understanding of your own needs, you can create a personal toolkit for navigating difficult situations. For example, the energizing qualities of a deadline can work to your advantage if properly harnessed.

Start with breathing. How do you breathe when you are angry? Shallow, quick breaths? How do you breathe when you cry? Probably irregularly. How do you breathe when you are relaxed and at ease? Likely slowly and with some level of comfort. Our breathing is linked with our internal experience, and by shifting breathing, we can shift thoughts and emotions. Breathing is among the few functions in the body that is simultaneously on auto-pilot but also voluntarily changeable. This means that you don't normally think about breathing; it's just happening to keep you alive. However, when you do pay attention to it, you can change the rate and rhythm of your breathing and even halt it for a period of time. As a result, by focusing on your breathing, you can change the nervous system response in the body. By slowing and regulating breathing patterns, we can engage a physical relaxation response that may shift negative emotions.[1, 2, 3]

For those times that you're seeking calm in a difficult situation, pay attention to your breathing. If you note that it is fast and irregular, try intentionally slowing it. A quick Google search will reveal multiple breathing techniques with timed in-breaths and out-breaths that promote relaxation. The overall goals of most techniques are to make the out-breath longer than the in-breath, really fill the lungs on the inhale and empty them on the exhale, and to pause between inhales and exhales.

▶ Try breathing in (through your nose if possible) for a count of 4–6 (one-one thousand, two-one thousand, three-one thousand...), pause for a count of 4–6, and then breathe out (also through your nose if possible) for a count of 6–8, pause for a count of 2. When done, repeat the cycle.

- Try to do this cyclical breathing for at least 15–30 seconds. Over time, build up time to what feels comfortable to you. As you continue to practice and gain comfort, slow the count down, giving yourself a little more time and a deeper in-breath and out-breath. Try to feel the air going in and going out. (Shelley: I focus on the sensation of the incoming cool air and outgoing warm air at the tip of my nostrils.)

- What do you notice about any physical sensations? Any emotional sensations?

Chapter 3

Wake-up Call

Everything you must know about sleep but were too tired to ask.

James Maas, PhD, author of *Sleep for Success*[1]

Should you feel drowsy and fall asleep while reading this chapter, we would not be surprised; many adults are sleep-deprived. A lack of sleep can throw life out of balance, and specifically impact how and what we eat. Studies have shown that people who are sleep-deprived snack more than those who are well rested. Some research suggests that sleep-deprived people may pick less nutritionally dense food because they are seeking a quick energy boost versus actually nourishing themselves.[2]

Adults need about 7–9 hours of sleep on a regular basis to function at their best,[3] yet many do not get sufficient sleep. If you're someone who has trouble falling asleep or staying asleep, or wakes up frequently in the middle of the night, you are not alone. In fact, chances are that if you're awake in the wee hours, so is your neighbor next door or across the street.

Unfortunately, teens also struggle with many of these same sleep issues and, in fact, are among the most sleep-deprived age group in the world![4] Most adolescents need close to nine hours of sleep per night (younger kids and athletes need even more), yet they average closer to six hours per night.

And yet both science and our own common sense tell us

that a good night's sleep is essential to our overall wellness. Adequate sleep affects mood, energy, academic and athletic performance, immune function, coordination, and alertness. It can even impact the frequency with which someone gets injured. Sleep is vital for physiological and psychological function as well as recovery. Sleep deprivation can be deadly for humans and have significant impacts on physical and cognitive function. It has been shown to have similarly devastating consequences to driving drunk. Drowsy driving is the number-one cause of death in teens.[5]

No doubt, you have seen your teen try to "catch up" on sleep during weekends or other down time. However, sleep is not as recoverable as you may think, and the idea of "sleep recovery" is a myth. Even if a person sleeps for a few extra hours on the weekend, this does not undo the negative effects of chronic lack of sleep during the week—specifically on attentiveness, short-term memory, school and work performance, accidents, and exam results to name a few.

Many people don't realize that they are not sleeping enough and adjust to a baseline of fatigue. Often, we accept that "tired" is normal and don't fully realize that fatigue is not normal until an experience or event forces a personal review. It's a little striking that "Saturday" or an equivalent occasion, such as a vacation or other downtime, is an event in our busy, sleep-deprived lives, in which we give our body what it needs. Additionally, 70 percent of surveyed parents think their teen is getting adequate sleep when in reality less than 15 percent actually are.[6] Ask your teen when they last felt rested and how many hours of sleep they got the night before. While you're at it, ask yourself the same question!

BENEFITS OF SLEEP

So, if you are feeling ready to talk sleep with your teen, establish firm-compassionate boundaries on what's non-negotiable.

Once you've assessed how you and your teen are sleeping, find a time to talk through what you've learned and strategize with your child about how to improve everyone's rest time. Self-identified goals are often more motivating than external rules. However, with the many demands of modern life, one approach with your teen may be to discuss their personal goals and educate them about how sleep helps them achieve these goals.

This approach offers a two-fold benefit, in that it gives you insight into what your teen finds valuable and also allows you to align with them in achieving their goals. Now, if your teen says their goal is to play video games until 1 a.m., that's not going to fly, and we fully support limit setting. However, if your teen indicates that their chosen sport is a highly important aspect of their life and that they need another hour at night to finish schoolwork, it's worth troubleshooting with them about how to "find" even 30 extra minutes in the day to decrease night-time schoolwork. Some motivators:

Improved Athletic Performance

Getting sufficient sleep can improve sports performance, literally overnight. The difference between winning and losing in competitive sports often comes down to milliseconds. A good night's rest can improve reaction time, which is the speed at which a person responds to a stimulus. This can translate to getting to the ball a little faster, making the tackle in time, crossing the finish line first, or otherwise gaining a powerful competitive edge.

Conversely, insufficient sleep slows reaction time significantly.[7] In fact, even pulling just one all-nighter can make our reaction time ten times slower.[8] Read that last sentence again. When swimmers extended their average sleep to ten hours a night, their reaction time decreased by 0.5 seconds (in other words, they swam faster).[9, 10] Similarly, when Stanford basketball players slept for ten hours, their reaction times also got quicker.[11] These athletes had more energy, improved overall performance, ran faster sprints, and their shooting accuracy improved. Accuracy is important in precision sports like baseball, golf, football, and any place where catching, throwing, hitting, and scoring matter. Can you think of a sport in which accuracy doesn't matter?

Sleep also improves split-second decision making, which can translate directly into fewer errors on the field. Better judgment yields fewer injuries and concussions. Adolescent athletes who slept less than eight hours a night were 1.7 times more likely to get injured.[12] During sleep, growth hormone is released, which helps with muscle growth and repair, making it an essential ingredient for recovery. Lebron James has been quoted as saying there is no better form of recovery than sleep (he gets close to 11 hours a night).[13]

Sleep also helps to consolidate learned skills into automatic muscle memory. The brain continues to learn even after practice ends. So, if you go to practice and then have a good night's rest, your brain is helping you improve while you sleep! Activity supports sleep and sleep supports activity. People who engage in regular physical activity also see benefits to their sleep, including longer sleep time, better sleep quality and structure, and less time awake at night.

Improved Mood

It has been well established that sleep affects mood and mood affects sleep. Dr. Meeta Singh is the service chief of sleep medicine, as well as section head and medical director, at the Henry Ford Sleep Help Center in Michigan. She states: "Sleep touches everything, but the effect on mental health is really profound. You can't really talk about mental health without giving sleep a seat at the table."[14]

Sleep disorders are often seen as a consequence of stress

or other medical and mental health diagnoses. However, we now know that many medical and mental health issues can be made worse by poor or insufficient sleep. So sleep isn't just linked to mental health because feeling unwell leads to poor sleep. It is fundamentally linked because if you don't sleep well, you're unlikely to feel well. Moods, as well as feelings of sadness, depression, and irritability, can be made more severe with insufficient or poor sleep. When we are tired, it can be more difficult to concentrate and complete tasks or engage in meaningful activities. In short: poor sleep may not be a by-product of a primary medical or mental health issue, but it could be a primary contributor that must be addressed as part of a therapeutic plan.

Most people agree that if they don't get enough sleep, they are, well, a bit cranky. A vicious cycle begins churning, in which the less someone sleeps, the worse they feel, and the worse they feel, the harder it is to sleep. The teens we see in our practice often describe feeling irritable; their parents describe them as moody. They yawn during sessions and describe an overall lack of energy. Late-night conversations, texting, and peer engagement are common parts of the adolescent experience. And we get it! A meaningful social life is an important and positive aspect of adolescence. But forgoing sleep in favor of night-time communication on a regular basis could have a negative impact on your child's health and mental health. Feelings of sadness, depression, and irritability can be made more severe with insufficient or poor sleep. It can be more difficult to concentrate and complete tasks or engage in meaningful activities. Talking to your teen about ways in which they can "call it" about how late they are engaging with friends may be a way to structure sleep and allow for more rest. Perhaps the ticket to having more pleasant interactions with your teen is finding a way to add back some of the hours of sleep we know they are missing.

Improved Immune Function

Sleep affects immunity and is a time of restoration for the body. A well-rested body is better equipped to fight infection or illness. During sleep, cytokines are released that fight infection; too little sleep lowers the amount of these cytokines and other immune cells. If you are getting less than six hours of sleep a night, you are four times more likely to catch a cold.[15]

Improved Academic Performance

Lack of sleep makes your brain foggy. A foggy mind isn't a helpful tool in school, life, sports, or most other things we care about. When school start times were shifted later, researchers found that SAT scores increased by a net of 212 points, truancy went down, and lateness went down just one year later.[16] Studies also show that those who are sleeping longer did better on math tests,[17] and those with better sleep efficiency (this assesses the quality and quantity of sleep by comparing the amount of actual sleep time with the total time spent in bed) did better in math and language subjects.[18]

Improved Connection to Hunger and Fullness Cues

A good night's sleep regulates hunger hormones (ghrelin) and satiety hormones (leptin), making it easier to eat in response to our body's wisdom. Lack of sleep can alter your hunger and satiety hormones, making it difficult to identify natural hunger cues and fullness. When we're sleep-deprived, we are less connected to our body. First, we may tend to eat mindlessly while tired, paying less attention to what we are choosing. Second, we may end up "feeding tired"—eating not for nutrition or pleasure, but for energy to stay awake.

Beauty Rest Is Real!

In a scientific study, participants were shown pictures of

individuals after a normal night's sleep and after being sleep-deprived. The same individual with eight hours of sleep was perceived as healthier and less tired, and even more attractive.[19] In another study, adults who slept seven to nine hours a night had skin that was more moisturized and could heal better after ultraviolet light exposure, compared with people who slept five hours per night.[20] Also, a lack of sleep can cause acne and lead to worse acne flares.[21] Sleep impacts every aspect of our health, including the appearance of health.

GOT RHYTHM? (SLEEP RHYTHM, THAT IS...)

Even though teens should be getting at least eight to nine hours of sleep a night (athletes about 9.25 hours), they are actually getting closer to seven hours, and often less than that. Sleep can be even more important in your teen years than at other stages of life. As we discuss in other chapters in this book, the teen years are a key growth time and sleep is a crucial aspect of healthy growth and development.

Our circadian rhythm is our "master clock." This internal clock is synchronized to our physical and emotional environment, the time zone in which we live, and our light and dark cues. Light during the day and darkness at night are needed to keep our circadian rhythm on schedule. This same rhythm influences many other biological functions, including hunger cues, satiety, and levels of fatigue.

Our sleep cycle (aka circadian rhythm) is genetic. You likely have at least one parent with the same circadian rhythm as yours. There is the early bird (early to bed and early to rise), a group somewhere in the middle, and the night owl (late to bed and late to wake). You may note that different children in your household or extended family have sleep patterns similar to one biological parent. You may also have noticed this for yourself.

As your child moves into their teenage years, their circadian rhythm shifts. Teens start to get tired later and wake up later. Parents may feel their child has become lazy, sleeping the day away. Parents may want to pull the sheets off their child, open the curtains, and force their teen out of bed. But this is how a teen brain is actually wired. There is a real biochemical change in the teen brain that changes the drive for bedtime and wake time. For adults, midnight might feel like the middle of the night, but for a teen, midnight might legitimately be too early with little biological sleep pressure. Teens stay up late and will keep busy during these late hours doing homework, hanging out with friends, or being on screens. Yet the demands of life, school, and other activities don't allow for teens to sleep in, and they still are required to be up early. This pattern causes teens to have a shortened night's sleep over and over again.

Sleeping late on weekends causes a circadian shift, making it hard to go back to the school schedule on Monday. Establishing a regular sleep/wake schedule each night helps teens to keep their circadian rhythms in, well, rhythm! Parents can help their teens create a healthy sleep schedule. Talk to your teen about a night-time routine to wind down, which can include having a "tech-free" window before bed, and initiating calming activities in low light.

SLEEP DISRUPTORS

Technology is part of our lives and has improved how we live, learn, and travel in the world. Overall, technology can be great, but tech has really impacted human sleep patterns. One of many reasons teens get less sleep is because of technology. The 2017 Youth Risk Behavior Study reported that those who were on screens more were more likely to have insufficient sleep than those who were on screens less.[22] Teens spend a mind-boggling nine hours per day on tech, with some 13-year-olds checking social media 100 times per day.[23] Nine hours is more than most teens are sleeping at night! The COVID-19 pandemic only increased time on screens, with activities that were typically offline (school day) also being completed partially or completely online.

Time on technology competes with sleep time and can be activating. Teens can struggle to go into the deeper stages of sleep because their mind is awake and waiting for that next text, update, or message. Teen FOMO (Fear of Missing Out) is high, and has been studied as it relates to sleep; one out of two teens check their phone in the middle of the night to see what they are missing. This is so disruptive that researchers are now working on FOMO-R (Fear of Missing Out Reduction) strategies for managing excessive cell phone use, which includes using auto-reply, filtering, and status checks. This also includes education on how FOMO occurs and skills on how to deal with it, such as self-talk and checklists.[24]

Even the light in our environment or emanating from our gadgets can stimulate our brain and keep us awake. Human sleep rhythms were previously synchronized with natural light cues, such as sunrise and sunset, but artificial light fundamentally changed our lives and our ability to stay awake and pursue tasks later into the evening and even late at night. This is problematic because light is a major disruptor of an important sleep hormone called melatonin. Melatonin helps us to fall asleep, and when our bodies and brains are too stimulated by light, melatonin secretion can be suppressed, disrupting our sleep. There are now apps that help to reduce the blue light in your computers, iPad, and phones for this very reason.

Blue-light glasses have been associated with a variety of benefits including less eye strain, reduction of eye disease, fewer headaches, and improved sleep. Some experts say it's not the blue light that is the problem, it's the digital overuse that is causing harm, but more research is needed.

A 2017 study by the University of Houston found that participants wearing blue-light glasses showed about a 58 percent increase in their night-time melatonin levels.[25] This helps improve sleep at night, despite being on devices during the day. These glasses are not regulated and range in price from tens to hundreds of dollars, though it's hard to know what you're getting. A market study report predicted that the global market for blue-light eyewear will increase to $27 million by 2024, up from $18 million in 2019.[26]

While it sounds promising, what would be even better would be to take the tech out of the bedroom and banish it to a charging station in the kitchen when it's time to sleep! If that's almost inconceivable, then stop and ask why? Why can't *we* put our tech away or why can't we ask our child to put it away too? What is so pressing that all of the detrimental effects of sleep deprivation make keeping the device next to us worth it?

Caffeine is another not-so-sneaky sleep disruptor. To really get enough sleep, it's important to watch caffeine consumption. Too much caffeine, timed incorrectly, can make it impossible to fall asleep. Caffeine is a stimulant and a widely available (coffee, tea, many chocolate-containing items, some medicines) substance that is classified as a "psychoactive drug".[27] Psychoactive drugs are "substances that, when taken in or administered into one's system, affect mental processes, e.g. perception, consciousness, cognition or mood and emotions."[28] Ingestion of caffeine can give a boost of energy, lead to increased heart rate or blood pressure, and can also disrupt the chemical signals that support and advance the urge to sleep.[29, 30] Research shows 75 percent of kids today are consuming caffeine, and the more caffeine someone consumes, the less sleep they get.[31] The half-life (the amount of time about half of the caffeine breaks down in the body) of caffeine is five to six hours, but this varies based on each person's caffeine metabolism. This means that if you have caffeine at 12 p.m., 50 percent of it is still in your system six hours later, and 25 percent is still coursing through your body at midnight.

We are seeing kids consuming caffeine in various forms, from coffee drinks to energy drinks, and doing this very late into the afternoon and night...and then not sleeping well. If your teen is struggling to fall asleep, stay asleep, waking up suddenly in the middle of the night, or is feeling anxious throughout the day, you might want to help them conduct a careful inventory of caffeinated products in their diet, including hidden sources of caffeine found in supplements, chocolate, bottled drinks and drinks from coffee houses.

It will require work to adjust how and when your teen takes in caffeine. Start with a conversation with your teen about how and when they are consuming their caffeine. Is it part of a social activity or are they trying to boost energy? Break down the specifics without judgment. If change is needed, then discuss changing types of products or the timing of consumption (push to early morning versus late afternoon). Switching to non-caffeinated options might help some transition off, but keep in mind that many decaffeinated products contain some caffeine or other stimulants. While this may be a difficult conversation, it will fundamentally help with overall health and well-being. Taking stock of personal habits in this way ultimately helps your teen to reach their goals.

The Buzz on Alcohol and Other Substances

Alcohol is the most commonly used substance among young people in the U.S.[32] In fact, according to the 2019

Youth Risk Behavior Survey, 29 percent of high school students had consumed alcohol in the past 30 days when surveyed.[33]. Among the many dangerous consequences of underage drinking (see the resource section at the end of the book for more information), alcohol can affect adolescent brain development, which can have lifelong effects.[34] As it pertains to sleep, alcohol will cause "sleep fragmentation," which will negatively affect REM sleep. REM (rapid eye movement) sleep is a stage of sleep where the brain is active. REM sleep is essential for memory, learning efficiency, and alertness.[35, 36, 37] A disruption to REM sleep will leave you feeling groggy. Although many say they fall "right to sleep" after drinking, don't mistake falling asleep quickly for high-quality rest.

Cannabis—better known in many cultures as marijuana, pot, weed, grass, 420, ganga, dope, herb, and many other names—is legal in an increasing number of states, yet it is currently illegal in all 50 states for minors. Legal or not, teens turn to marijuana for a variety of reasons, some of which include to help with sleep or as a tool for managing anxiety, depression, pain, and/or migraines. Cannabis use has been shown to have negative effects, such as increasing sleepiness during the day and causing withdrawal symptoms such as irritability and insomnia.[38] Interestingly, a recent study showed that those who smoked cannabis as a teen were more likely to have insomnia later in life.[39] A possible explanation? A growing body of literature suggests that exposure to cannabis during key developmental years may lead to short- and long-term changes in brain development and function.[40, 41, 42]

Additionally, the use of other nicotine-containing substances, such as cigarettes or chewing tobacco, can also disrupt sleep. Nicotine is a stimulant, which will make you feel alert and awake, even when you might really be tired. Those who try to quit smoking are likely to experience a variety of symptoms, such as headaches, irritability, anxiety, and, yes, sleepless nights.

Mitsuko, a 17-year-old female, was smoking nicotine using a vape. She had a lot of energy during the day but her parents noted she was also sleeping a lot during the day. After sharing with her doctor that she was vaping, the doctor felt the nicotine was causing a false sense of wakefulness during the day, then a crash. The naps were dysregulating her sleep at night, causing her to feel tired during the day. She then felt she "needed" the nicotine to stay awake—a vicious cycle. Weaning off the nicotine, eliminating midday naps, allowed her to go to bed at night and sleep through the night.

SLEEP MEDICATIONS

Before turning to sleep medicine for you or your teen, it's first important to explore the possible reasons for the sleep disruption. CBT-I (cognitive behavioral therapy for insomnia) is the first line of treatment before starting medications. With CBT-I, trained professionals teach you how to tackle your sleep issues, reduce sleep anxiety, and improve the quality of sleep. A few things to try first include: changing the amount or timing of caffeine you or your teen are consuming, reducing screen time, wearing blue-light glasses, and adding meditation and/or a breathwork program.

Sleep medicines should be assessed by a medical doctor and ideally by a sleep specialist. Medications can be addicting and are not meant for long-term use. The brain can get used to medications and, over time, might require larger doses to get the same effect. They can also cause daytime side effects including drowsiness and trouble concentrating. Some of the medications on the market for sleep can cause even more significant side effects, such as sleep walking, sleep talking, or even driving without knowledge of doing so. As a result, some of these medications have what's called a "black box warning." Additionally, these medications do not induce a natural sleeping state. They sedate you, which does not provide the same sense of restfulness.

More than three million Americans take melatonin, according to the U.S. National Center for Health Statistics. Melatonin can help you to fall asleep, but not necessarily to stay asleep. Melatonin is best for those wishing to fall asleep earlier than their current bedtime (if you are a night owl) or for those struggling with jet lag. Melatonin is a supplement, so it is not regulated by the FDA. A study done in Canada looked at how much melatonin was in a variety of melatonin supplements and found that some contained less than 83% to 478% the amount stated on the label. Eight of the 31 melatonin supplements screened contained significant quantities of the drug serotonin, which is used to treat neurological disorders.[43, 44] In other words, caution is needed when taking unregulated supplements.

WAYS TO IMPROVE SLEEP

Sleep hygiene is your routine for taking care of your body's sleep needs. How attentive are you to listening to the cues when you are feeling tired? Getting yourself off to bed on time and up again at a regular time is an acquired skill and one that is likely to enhance your life by improving your mood, preventing disconnected eating, and boosting performance and focus.

- Establish a regular sleep schedule. The key to regular, restorative sleep is consistency. Parents can help guide and enforce a consistent sleep schedule. This means committing to going to bed around the same time every night and waking up around the same time every morning, even on weekends.

- Create a wind-down routine. This is an important way to train your body to get ready for a good night's sleep. It is a repeated ritual that starts about an hour before bedtime. This routine is the signal that tells your body it is time to relax and prepare for sleep. Activities during this time should not be stimulating, but they should be enjoyable! Think of things that support sleepiness, such as herbal tea, soothing music, a treasured blanket, some lavender oil next to your bed.

- Avoid drinking fluids right before bed and go to the bathroom before you get into bed, to avoid or minimize middle-of-the-night washroom visits. Let's all say it together now: if you're peeing, you're not sleeping! So build in a bathroom break to allow yourself uninterrupted rest to the greatest extent possible.

- Get continuous sleep. It's not okay to sleep four hours at night and four hours after school. That doesn't lead to high-quality restorative sleep. As much as possible, plan for seven to nine hours in a row.

- If you want to nap, choose a "power nap," which is a quick 30-minute nap. Avoid long naps, which will disrupt night-time sleep, making it hard for you to fall or stay asleep. It's like taking the lid off a pressure cooker. If your teen has to nap, a quick nap should do the trick. Set an alarm, and for sleepier teens, have them leave the alarm on the other side of the room so they actually have to get out of bed to turn it off.

- Aim to have a dark, cool, uncluttered room.

- Reduce light at night. Using smartphones, tablets, and computers at night can stimulate your brain and even suppress melatonin, making it harder to fall asleep. To block these cues, try using orange-tinted glasses or apps that reduce the blue lights from devices.

- Hold the phone! This will not make us popular, but it's a good idea to have a charging station somewhere in the house other than in your teen's bedroom. See the "Digital Agreements" section in Chapter 10 to encourage your teen to make agreements with their friends—for example, they could make a group agreement to be offline after 8 p.m. on school nights. Teens often rely on each other in the wee hours of the night, but this is not a healthy way to provide support for each other, given the drawbacks of sleep deprivation.

- Assess caffeine consumption. Is your child consuming caffeine, and if so, how much and when? Caffeine can stay in the system for a long time and can be disruptive to sleep. Can your child cut out caffeine? Reduce it? Shift the timing to earlier in the day?

- Aim to reduce substance use, especially right before bed. This includes alcohol, cannabis, chewing tobacco, and cigarettes.

- Try not to exercise right before bed. Activity wakes the body up and can keep you physiologically stimulated. The heart rate can remain elevated for a long time and cause the body to remain alert when you'd like to be winding down and relaxing.

- Keep the bed for sleep. Don't do homework, eat, or use tech in bed. Allow the mind to relax and associate the bed with sleep and rest, not work, homework, snacks, or socializing.

- Parents and caregivers should practice—and even more importantly, model—the above recommendations. Children and teens soak in their environment and are more likely to repeat behaviors and patterns that are familiar.

If you have followed all of the above suggestions but still can't get to sleep after 25–30 minutes, get up and out of bed. Your bed should be associated with restful sleep. Think of it this way: you'd never sit at a dinner table just waiting to get hungry. After the 30-minute mark, get out of bed and read with a dim light, meditate, do light yoga stretches, do artwork, and return when you begin to feel sleepy. According to Dr. Matthew Walker, author of *Why We Sleep*, "Lying awake in bed hoping to fall asleep is like trying to remember someone's name you forgot... the harder you try the worse it is."[45]

SLEEP DISORDERS

One of the reasons many people think they have insomnia is that they are going to bed earlier than their body is ready for sleep. For example, if genetically you are a night owl and you try to fall asleep at 9 p.m., it may have more to do with your circadian rhythm than your willpower. If that is not the case, and you suspect you truly have insomnia, then the CBT-I techniques mentioned earlier in this chapter will likely not work. The Insomnia Severity Index is a tool you can use before talking with a professional.[46]

Sometimes there are medical reasons that explain why someone is not able to sleep well. We are not going to review every one of these conditions, but we do feel that it is important for you to know that disorders such as sleep apnea (not being able to breathe well while sleeping and more common among snorers) or narcolepsy (excessive daytime sleepiness, sometimes with sudden episodes of falling asleep or "sleep attacks") among others, can lead to excessive fatigue and very dysregulated sleep. Chronic health conditions such as asthma, depression, and diabetes can also cause sleep problems. If you feel that you or your teen have tried several sleep hygiene suggestions but are still struggling to sleep, it may be time to talk with a professional.

EXPLORATION: Wind-down Routines

Stretch your body and imagine some sleepy sheep. We're going to help you create your wind-down routine! Night-time is a time of reception, not reflection. Some of our favorite additions to the routine include a hot shower, knitting, sewing, reading, stretching, yoga, meditation, breath work, writing, or journaling.[47]

One hour before bed, I commit to doing these relaxing wind-down activities:

_____

_____

_____

_____

EXPLORATION: Worry Journal

About an hour before you go to bed, write down anything that has been bothering you throughout the day. Believe it or not, this simple act has been shown to have a therapeutic effect. Cathartic self-help techniques allow us to access the emotions or worries we have stored from our day and release them. We suggest a "free-write" style of writing. Set a timer for, say, five minutes and write nonstop during the time allotted for the exercise. The idea is to clear everything that is on your mind and get it out on paper. It's not healthy to keep your frustrations pent up inside, nor is it healthy to regenerate them over and over again, past the point of getting any new information. After your timer goes off, make a commitment to put your worries on the metaphorical shelf.

Chapter 4

The Young and the Restless

BUST A MOVE

Exercise is a fun way to express yourself and share different aspects of your personality or qualities that others don't usually get to see. For example, colleagues at work may not get to see the more competitive side of you, the one that dives for the ball on the court and gives your all to make the shot. They may not see the Zen side that shows up in the yoga class and peaces out during Savasana. Clients tell us that it's refreshing to see a different side of themselves reflected back through sports and the many enriching aspects of activity, such as competition, teamwork, engagement, discipline, and joyful movement, to name just a few.

While athletics and intense exercise may not be for everyone, some level of regular activity is generally a positive. During exercise, endorphins (hormones) are released which can provide what's known as an "all-natural high." This feeling can last several hours after exercise is finished. It might initially be challenging to incorporate more intentional movement into your life or your teen's life if you have not done so in the past. However, many people indicate that they notice benefits after beginning a regular exercise program. Exercise has been shown to improve mood, reduce stress, improve sleep, improve attention in school, and support emotional regulation. Interestingly, research has also shown that we are all more likely to live a longer, healthier life if we include physical activity.[1] Our bodies come in all different shapes and sizes, and rather than focusing on weight to improve health, long-term health and wellness can be enhanced through regular and engaging physical activity that is enjoyable.

In this chapter, we discuss the benefits of exercise, as well as our individual relationships with activity, exercise avoidance, and even the supposed morality inherent in moving. We review several barriers that can make it difficult to establish a pleasurable movement schedule.

THE BENEFITS OF MOVING

- Improves mood, makes you happy.

- Keeps emotions stable.

- Reduces stress, clears cortisol.

- Improves concentration.

- Helps with sleep.

- Improves body image.

- Strengthens your heart, muscles, and tendons.

- Fine-tunes your hunger/satiety cues.

- Improves coordination.

- Gives a sense of self-mastery.

- Increases ability to learn and retain new information.

- Provides an opportunity to try out new activities.

- Is an opportunity to socialize with others.

- Helps us become aware of, and adjust, our effort/intensity.

- Builds the immune system, decreasing the likelihood of injury or illness.

- Allows for personal growth and learning through creating and practicing new skills that may be challenging or out of the norm for you, such as boxing or fencing, or even aerial silks (ooh la la!).

TAKE THE MORALITY OUT OF MOVING

There is an insidious, not-often-talked-about morality associated with moving. You're "good" if you have exercised that day and "bad" if you haven't. These types of judgments create pressure and promote narrow ideas of what it means to be healthy or fit. Within those narrow ideas are value judgments about someone's inherent worth, with those that prioritize athleticism being "better" than those who do not. Unfortunately, "better" is often equated with thinness and an athletic body is immediately associated with well-defined muscles or six-pack abs and a "cut" physique. According to the Women's Sports Foundation, 40 percent of teen girls are not participating in sports, and they are also two times more like than boys to drop out of sports by age 14.[2] Reasons include feeling awkward and not liking the way they look, according to research.[3]

As we take in and then transmit these values, many of us fall victim to limited notions of personal wellness as they relate to movement. Unfortunately, many of these same messages also include layers of social and gender bias ("you run like a girl" or the perception that members of some ethnic groups are better or worse at certain sports). This pressure to move—or to move in a specific way—has the opposite effect, and can negatively affect sports performance and play. When talking to teens, it is critical that parents support their teens in achieving their physical goals, while emphasizing joyful activity that is aligned with true health.

Exercising to burn calories, lose weight, or alter one's appearance creates an unhealthy relationship with movement. Linking exercise to food intake in any way—"I ate so much today, so I'm going to go exercise"—teaches kids that they should compensate for food consumed with exercise, which is a dangerous and disturbing message that, over time, can potentially lead to the development of an eating disorder.

Be mindful of your own intentions for your child's exercise; if you feel judgmental about your child's weight, when you tell them to exercise, they may have your number and know that your request is really "you just want me to exercise so I can lose weight." Studies show that exercise doesn't facilitate weight loss anyway. It turns out, after starting an exercise program, most people increase what they eat, or generally move less in other areas of their life, off-setting the energy deficit they created from exercise.[4] Promising someone they will lose weight if they exercise may be the quickest way to end their relationship with moving, and set up destructive practices, such as exercising for weight loss instead of overall health. Instead, parents can focus on the many practical benefits of exercise, including improved mood, energy, and sleep, stress relief, and metabolic fitness.

Choose What Moves You

Different types of movement help to strengthen bones, build muscle, and help with flexibility. There are so many ways to move, beyond just playing team sports. Your child does not have to be a soccer, baseball, or tennis star to get moving. Parents can help their kids cultivate curiosity about what activities, if any, interest them. Fun ideas include gardening, paddle boarding, mowing the lawn, water aerobics, hide and seek, flying kites, Pilates, roller skating, scavenger hunts, yoga, Zumba, skateboarding, rock climbing, hiking, shoveling snow, playing Just Dance, and more!

What movement inspires you? What movement do you like to do as a family?

IS THERE SUCH A THING AS TOO MUCH EXERCISE?

In a society that praises exercise, applauds thinness, and overly focuses on "health" (diet culture), the reality that people *can* exercise too much must be addressed. It is common to hear parents express that they want their children to be more physically active. Unfortunately, it is also common for youth, particularly impressionable or more concrete youth, to take "health" messages to an extreme. Exercising in a balanced way means participating in a variety of enjoyable activities while taking into consideration the other responsibilities in one's life. Sport psychologist Riley Nickols calls this "balanced exercise," and reminds us of a very important question: "Do you structure your life around exercise or training for your sport, or do you structure exercise and training for your sport around life?"

Parents should be on the lookout for signs of over-exercise and whether their active teen is sufficiently fueling and maintaining nutritional intake for their level of activity.

Chloe is a 15-year-old who increased her exercise during the pandemic after team sports were canceled. Formerly a competitive soccer player, she started bike riding and running several times a week to "stay fit." Her parents noticed that she was always tired, was more irritable and moody, and had no energy. When she saw her doctor, it was determined her heart rate was dangerously low and her vital signs were unstable (explaining why she was always dizzy). Plus, her menstrual cycle was delayed, suggesting hormone changes and dysregulation.

At first glance, an increase in activity may appear to be a positive, but excessive exercise with unbalanced eating can cause serious health effects that warrant attention and monitoring from a medical health professional.

Too much exercise, in the absence of appropriate caloric intake, can be dangerous and can also come with a notable decline in performance (a coach may even spot this first). Sufficient nutritional intake (food and fluids) drives all bodily functions, and without adequate nutrition, especially for prolonged periods, an individual will experience negative physical, emotional, and cognitive changes. Your child might be physically slower, weaker, tired, and more prone to injury, and may not make progress in their sport despite intense training. They may be more irritable, express feelings of depression, and exhibit decreased endurance. This is incongruent with their initial goals of achieving health and excelling at their sport. Instead, they are experiencing the negative consequences of dysregulated activity that is not balanced with a self-nourishing practice. Researchers have given a name to this energy imbalance as it pertains to athletes: "RED-S," which stands for Relative Energy Deficiency in Sports.[5]

Exercising too much, especially without eating enough to cover the activity, can also cause life-threatening medical complications, which can affect many systems of the body, including the heart. Failure to increase one's intake to account for movement can result in abnormalities in heart rate and blood pressure, hormone suppression (estrogen and testosterone), reductions in bone density leading to stress fractures, gastrointestinal changes such as slowing leading to constipation and pain, and much more. This can happen to anyone, even those who appear to be healthy athletes, and is directly related to the energy imbalances of excess exercise and insufficient nutrition.

SIGNS YOUR TEEN HAS A BALANCED RELATIONSHIP WITH EXERCISE

- They are able to listen to their body and respond appropriately. This might result in feeling up to moving some days and feeling as though rest is needed on other days.

- They participate in activities with internal goals, such as the expectation of fun, versus external goals, such as weight loss.

- They actually *like* the activity they're doing.

- They see exercise as flexible, meaning that they adjust their workouts when school, social, or family commitments arise.

- They allow their body to rest, knowing that rest will not diminish their desire to exercise on other days.[6]

- They enjoy their rest time.

- They eat and enjoy food and adequately fuel their level of activity.

- They change up their exercise with the seasons—for example, in the rainy season they may increase yoga and decrease soccer/hiking.

There is also "unbalanced exercise." The warning signs may be more obvious or visible to others. Or your internal sense that things are off may be triggered, signaling time to pause and reflect if the current practice is working for your teen.

SIGNS YOUR TEEN MAY HAVE AN UNBALANCED RELATIONSHIP WITH EXERCISE

- They feel anxious if they don't get to do their workout on a particular day.

- They think of working out as a way to make up for what they ate.

- They work out even when they are sick, injured, or tired.

- They are working out to delay or modify physical changes to their body.

- They work out for external goals only (chiefly, physical appearance).

- They work out in odd places at odd times.

- They don't eat enough for the energy they are expending.

- Family or friends have expressed concern that they are exercising too much.

- They force themselves to exercise even when they do not feel like doing so.

- They forgo previously enjoyable social or family

gatherings as a result of their workout schedule or the urge to exercise.

To assess if your teen has an unbalanced relationship with exercising, feel free to check out the Compulsive Exercise Test.[7] If you find that several of these warning signs apply to your child, we recommend that you consult with a weight-inclusive, non-diet registered dietitian, therapist, and/or doctor, in order to better understand your child's relationship with exercise and to explore how your child might be able to become more flexible and spontaneous.

EXPLORING BARRIERS TO EXERCISE

Okay, message received: there are a multitude of benefits to moving our bodies regularly and joyfully. However, some individuals have difficulty consistently incorporating physical activity, while others avoid it entirely.

There are many reasons why an individual might abstain from moving, including:

- Fell out of the habit.

- Not finding enjoyment in exercise.

- Feeling uncomfortable moving in their body.

- Fear of teasing or fat stigma from others (avoiding activity in an effort not to be judged).

- Equipment that doesn't accommodate different-sized bodies.

- Self-conscious in gym clothes.

- Can't find clothes that fit.

- Lack of confidence or experience in trying out new activities.

- Unsure what exercises to do or how to do them.

- Low energy or mood (depression, anxiety).

- Lack of safe places to play or exercise.

- Being a person with disabilities, requiring safe and specific spaces or equipment.

GET IN THE GROOVE

For those who have been avoiding exercise, it's important to reflect on the specifics that may be limiting you or your teen. For example, if your teen needs help developing skills, or needs support with overcoming fears around trying a new skill, then the primary need is likely support and understanding. Avoidance of a particular activity can maintain fear of it. Consider the Goldilocks approach, in which the goal is to find an activity that is not "too hot" (trying out for the NFL) or "too cold" (no activity at all), but instead one that is "just right" (walks or shooting hoops at the local court!).

Challenging your child may cause an initial increase in anxiety, but the good news is that a process called habituation occurs over time. Imagine how a child feels the first time they timidly slide into the deep end of the pool. At first, it's scary, and they may have to force themselves to stay put; after some time and support, the deep waters seem more manageable. Through repeated effort, reassurance, and practice, your child will likely evolve from a timid toe-dipper to a cannon-baller. By reframing this as a challenge, and using consistent encouragement, this same stress response can turn into joy and pride after achieving a new goal and overcoming a fear.

It's easy to get out of the habit of moving, and if that's the case, consider using research-based interventions on the latest neuroscience of habit. Dr. Joanna Steinglass from Columbia

Center for Eating Disorders states that if you are looking to increase your habit of exercise, first consider ways to make it easier to do, and find the things that feel good about doing it. For example, if you feel inspired to play more tennis, pick the time that best works into your schedule, that you could repeat regularly. If you naturally wake up at 9 a.m. on weekends, and you set your alarm to play tennis at 6 a.m., that early morning wake-up will eventually stop feeling comfortable, and the plan is likely to fizzle. Second, set up external cues in your environment while initiating your new habit. For example, put your tennis racket where you can see it before you crawl under the covers at night, and right where you can see it when you wake up. It'll be waiting for you in the morning! Finally, make sure you pay attention to what you enjoy about the new routine. You may not get the pleasure you are used to from sleeping late, so you need to make sure you attend to the sights and smells of the morning—or the fun of seeing your friend first thing in the morning—that you get from your new routine. Give that new reward plenty of air time. Try to sample different types of movement until you find the one you really enjoy. This is called joyful movement.[8]

B. Timothy Walsh of the Columbia Center for Eating Disorders notes that once behaviors become linked together into a routine, and once the chain of action is initiated, the rest follows with little mental effort.[9] Sometimes, however, habits take hold when they are not useful. If you are trying to break a bad habit, that's called "habit reversal." Creating a new habit is called "habit formation." Habit formation is the process by which new behaviors become automatic. If your teen feels inclined to lace up her tennis shoes and hit the courts as soon as they get home from school, they've acquired a habit. It takes a lot of effort to create a new automatic habit, but if you persist, it will become effortless, just like brushing your teeth.

Let's take a typical case. Your child used to love playing competitive soccer, but got burnt out or decided to take a break.

Fast-forward a couple of years: suddenly your teen's soccer passion is back! You wouldn't want them to go from limited movement for two years to rejoining the soccer team next week. However, we do suggest you consult with a knowledge-able parent, coach, or professional and create a safe plan that allows you to increase their activity (and intake) in a gradual manner, until they reach their goals. This will likely require what we call "action precedes motivation." In other words, don't wait to get in the mood to move—move first, to get you in the mood.

Once your teen is on the move, how do you help them *keep* moving? First, encourage them to explore their last frame of reference of movement. Was soccer something they really enjoyed, or, in the end, were they doing it for their coach? If they really didn't like it, it's important to explore different types of exercise, to see what they feel pulled to do. Some people would rather hand-shell 10,000 walnuts than go on a run. The monotonous nature of running or the discomfort the body might feel from continually pounding the pavement can be understandable deterrents for some. However, these same individuals may jump at the chance to play a pick-up basket-ball game or hike in the woods. A team sport may be more motivating for social teens. Or a hike in the woods with quiet time or scenic views may be most enjoyable and sustainable. In short, take the time to help your teen find a form of exercise they love and want to experience again and again.

Wendy had a client who wanted to start moving more, but she was so annoyed by her father's nonstop badgering about exercise that it almost had the opposite effect. In spite of her genuine, personal desire to be active, she and her father were unable to disengage from the power struggle. It was a lose-lose situation for both of them. After some time, and with guidance, the client was able to cultivate an enjoyment for moving that was entirely her own, rather than formed to appease her father.

She was able to reignite her passion for being active. This raises an important point: exercise burnout with kids is not typically from the sport, exercise, or movement itself, but from being forced to do it.

Other factors that impact movement are access to safe spaces. Some families live in locations that are not designed to promote movement—no bike lanes or easily accessible local parks—or in areas where activity outside may not be possible, such as unsafe neighborhoods. In these circumstances, parents and kids will have to be more intentional about picking places where they can be active. They may have to plan the hours or times of day that they visit recreational areas, such as remote hiking trails or courts in nearby neighborhoods. This need to overcome logistical barriers can be time-consuming. Fatigue after a long day, school, or work can all impact willingness to do anything extra, much less initiate exercise. This requires parents and teens to get creative and take stock of what is doable, feasible, and enjoyable. The simplest solution may be to turn on some music and dance until you sweat in the privacy of your home or room. Other options might be simple stretches or yoga poses. There has also been an influx of virtual exercise options in recent years, from online coaching, training, strength training, or sports classes, which might provide a viable solution. Parents and teens can brainstorm what's practical and realistic when time, energy, or access is limited.

Culturally, athleticism is considered the domain of the thin. Dr. Riley Nickols shares:

> Sports science research over the past few decades has shown that there are a multitude of factors that have been directly linked to impact athletic performance that often are minimized and neglected in lieu of weight, such as sleep, mental toughness, concentration, confidence, reaction time, rest, coordination, commitment, and coachability.

Things like skills training, endurance, flexibility, whether the athlete missed a meal, hydration, and following recovery protocols also impact sport performance, too—and this list can go on! Yet there continues to be a harmful, unnecessary, overemphasis on weight—which is just one of many factors affecting sport performance.

Dr. Nickols says:

> Forcing your body to reach a weight that is unnatural for your body can be harmful to your health, can suppress metabolism, and can result in unstable vital signs. Sport performance can also subsequently worsen as a result of being at an inappropriate weight through decrements in strength, power, speed while inhibiting the body's ability to recover while training. Our bodies and brain perform optimally at a weight that is individualized, and most appropriate for our unique genetic make-up, rather than attempting to modify weight to fit a perceived ideal.

Children and teens often experience criticism and even bullying simply for living at a higher weight. The assumption that they are inherently unhealthy and less skillful at their sport tends to go hand in hand with these attitudes. Unfortunately, but understandably, facing "fatphobia" can be debilitating and lead to exercise avoidance. Fatphobia is a term used to describe irrational discrimination and aversion towards those who are in larger bodies. Fatphobia may present itself as support or accolades for the larger-bodied person, where the guiding principles are that exercise is a means to an end for the more desired outcome—weight loss and thinness. Oppressive messages of stigma are omnipresent at home, in the workplace, on the playground, in popular images, songs, and films, and in the media. Stigma can increase feelings of shame, self-consciousness, and even guilt for just being oneself. This is demoralizing, and, further, is linked with chronic stress and its associated negative health impacts. Culturally, we are bombarded with the collective message that the only goal of a fat-bodied person is, or at least should be, to lose weight. The morality of weight loss and the glorification of thinness clearly (and falsely!) communicate that a fat body is wrong and needs to change.

Using the Word "Fat"

Aaron Flores, a fat-positive, non-diet registered dietitian who specializes in intuitive eating, Health at Every Size®, and helping clients reclaim Body Trust®, discussed his lived experience with the word "fat" in an episode of Signe's podcast *Therapy Rocks!*[10] He says:

> Using the word "fat" is a reclamation tool: "I'm going to reclaim this word and take some of the power out of it." I think that's exactly why I started doing it, and it's been an evolution to do that. There's so much fatphobia and weight bias in our world that the word fat has a lot of power to it, and we don't just mean fat when we say it, we mean a lot of other words behind it that are quite shaming and judgmental. So, when we hear that word, we're not just hearing the word fat. We're thinking of all the other things that are associated with it.
>
> For me, I started to use the word, and was like, "I wonder if I start using it more, does it become less powerful? Does it become less of a shame-driven word?" And now when I use it in talks or just in conversations with people, I notice they are very uncomfortable when they hear someone refer to themselves as fat. Not in some sort of self-deprecating way, just like, "I have brown hair, I have brown eyes, I'm wearing long pants and a sweater vest, and I'm fat." People will make comments: "C'mon, Aaron, no you're not." I'm like, yes I

> am. We don't need to sugar-coat it. I'm fat and I'm okay with it. It's my body, I get to decide how I want to refer to it, and it's actually given me a lot of pride in my body that might not have ever been there before.

Negative assumptions about the physical abilities, health habits, enthusiasm for movement, and even general personhood of fat people are woven into the fabric of many communities. This is particularly apparent in sports or group exercise activities, in which the facilitators may believe that larger-bodied students need more help or are less capable. Speaking about this on a podcast, Ragen Chastain, author of the popular blog Dances With Fat, shared that she was singled out because *she is fat* by the instructor during a dance class, despite having danced her whole life.

"Did my knees text you?" she quipped, describing her lived experience with this stigma.[11] She added:

Think about the times when you don't feel like going to the gym... Think about if going to the gym also meant people were also going to be absolutely cruel to you. How would you make time to go, and how much easier would it be to just skip it, even though it is something you would like to do if it was a positive situation?

Before pushing your child to go to the gym, explore if the gym you're considering is the right fit. Is the gym a supportive and safe place for a person with a different body shape, size, or ability? Do they have equipment that is usable for people of varying abilities and needs? Are staff members trained to be inclusive and non-discriminatory to larger-bodied folks and those with disabilities or other needs? Are group classes considerate of different skill levels, with instructors who can work with and guide a diverse clientele? Should you find a suitable gym, you may also want to check in with your child to see if they have clothing to move in that feels comfortable

If finding a gym is challenging, here are some weight-inclusive virtual training and movement options:

- **Joyn** offers joyful movement classes for adults and kids in larger bodies. Their site is about choice and body autonomy, and they ask their customers questions like "Would moving from a chair feel more supportive?" and "Would it feel better to slow down and meditate?" Their website features people of color and people of different sizes, and they offer fat-positive dance classes, yoga, chair movement, and more. **www.joyn.co**

- The **Big Fit Girl** app offers both seated and standing options, and a range of workouts with various types of equipment for all bodies. **https://fitnessapp.bigfitgirl.com**

- In **Fat Kid Yoga Club**, Marc Settembrino, a fat-queer yoga practitioner, has created inclusive yoga classes that are accessible to every body, regardless of size, shape, age, strength, or flexibility. **https://fatkidyogaclub.com**

- **Decolonizing Fitness** was founded by Ilya who is a black transmasculine person. The site focuses on "trans and body liberation, fat acceptance, disability, healing and racial justice." **www.patreon.com/DecolonizingFitness**

- **Fat Kid Dance Party** was founded by its creator, Bevin, after years of bullying. "Have you ever been called 'too much,' 'too fat' or felt too awkward to dance? Me too! After being bullied about my weight and my flamboyance as a kid, I never felt like I could dance in front of people." All sizes and bodies are welcome! www.fatkiddanceparty.com

- **Body Positive Fitness** helps people to feel happy with who they are and encourages clients to work out to be stronger, faster, more energetic, and all the other amazing benefits that come from moving your body that have nothing to do with changing your appearance. Their studio offers virtual classes and they work from a Health at Every Size® lens. www.bodypositivefitness.ca

- **FreetoBFit** is a body-affirming, safe space for all levels of movement, created to celebrate all the amazing things that our bodies can do. They encourage community, listening to your body needs, challenging your notions of what you can/can't do, and enjoying the way movement makes you feel—in the moment and long term. They are based in Seattle, but also offer virtual classes. https://freetobfit.com

- **Everybody Los Angeles** is devoted to creating and supporting a brave and inclusive environment for all bodies to move, strengthen, and heal. They feel that health and wellness should be accessible, affordable, and adaptive to all people regardless of their gender, size, age, ethnicity, or ability. Virtual classes are an option. www.everybodylosangeles.com

Exercising with Disabilities

According to the Centers for Disease Control, "A disability is any condition of the body or mind (impairment) that makes it more difficult for the person with the condition to do certain activities (activity limitation) and interact with the world around them (participation restrictions)."[12] A disability can be physical, cognitive, psychosocial, communicative, or sensory.[13] UNICEF estimates that 150 million children under 18 live with disabilities.[14] Those with disabilities might face weight stigma, as well as many challenges with moving joyfully. Talking with a physician or movement specialist can help those with disabilities find movement that works with their body and supports their needs.

Parents can talk to their teen and discuss if, how, when, and/or where their teen wants to participate in activity. Then parents can be their child's best advocate at school, in gyms, in classes, and so on. Does your child need specialized equipment, instruction, or both? Additionally, here are some at-home exercise ideas for those with disabilities:

- The **National Center on Health, Physical Activity and Disability** has videos for kids and adults and includes options for all abilities. They feature adapted yoga, wheelchair softball, theraband work, and more. **www.nchpad.org/Videos**

- **Adaptive Adventures** provides ongoing programs, camps, and clinics in cycling, climbing, kayaking, paddle boarding, dragon boat racing, skiing, snowboarding, water skiing, wakeboarding, and rafting, and serves over 30 states, Puerto Rico, and Canada each year. Their vision is for all individuals with physical disabilities to have access to participation in outdoor sports, regardless of their location, equipment needs, or economic status. **https://adaptiveadventures.org**

- **The Special Olympics website** provides resources for developing endurance, strength, stamina, and balance at home for athletes of all abilities. The Special Olympics site also provides additional resources for helping to support a child's transition to Special Olympics participation, competition management, coaching, and more. **https://resources.specialolympics.org/health/fitness/fit-5**

BODY AWARENESS

Now we invite you to explore your own body awareness. Our hope is that by taking the time to think about the answers to the questions here, you can help your teen develop a simple and streamlined way to make a decision to move or not. We don't want you to force your teen to move. Instead, we encourage you to work with them to find enjoyable and sustainable activities. And if they "choose" not to participate in regular activity, that's okay, too. Keeping communication open and periodically checking in may be more productive.

If you have concerns about health habits, then that's worth a discussion with your child, doctor, and/or other members of your support community. We encourage you to be mindful about how you approach the subject; don't assign value or morality to the situation at hand. Avoid statements such as "You're being lazy" or "You're gaining weight and you need to move." Instead, try "I'm wondering how you're doing and wanted to check in with you about (fill in the blank)." To get you started, here is a sample body awareness exploration. Use ours, or create your own, for personal use or to share with your teen.

I. What type of movement inspires you versus tires you today?

Going to yoga. It's warm. I like my instructor and their voice is so calming! Yikes, the thought of soccer practice is making me tired. It's cold outside and I don't want to run up and down the field today. I like warm, more calming, indoor activities.

2. How was your sleep last night?

   Less than 7 hours. A little restless. Would definitely prefer more rest and a couple more hours.

3. How would you describe your energy level?

   Energy level is a little low, probably because I had less than 7 hours of sleep last night.

4. How is your mood?

   Mood is off, I feel a bit "meh" today. I think doing some exercise may help. Yoga's my thing, so I'll start with that and see how long I last. I'm going to hop into bed earlier today!

5. Are you able to adjust, modify, or skip a planned workout if needed?

   Yes, I wouldn't do it if I was tired.

6. What type of movement would be joyful to you today?

   Restorative yoga. Walking maybe. I could dance a little.

EXPLORATION

1. What type of movement inspires you versus tires you today?

   _____

   _____

2. How was your sleep last night?

3. How would you describe your energy level?

4. How is your mood?

5. Are you able to adjust, modify, or skip a planned workout if needed?

6. What type of movement would be enjoyable for you today?

Chapter 5

Diet-free Parenting

Co-written by Anna Lutz, MPH, RD, LDN, CEDRD-S

Parents are taught that, in order to be a good parent, their child needs to eat a wide variety of "healthy" foods (kale and quinoa, anyone?), move their bodies in prescriptive ways, and be a certain size. This pressure can be passed on to children, leading to the absolute opposite of the desired effect. Restrictive feeding and weight talk in the home interfere with children's ability to listen to hunger and fullness cues, which can lead to overeating. Dieting and a focus on weight lead to increased weight, eating disorders, anxiety, and depression. Furthermore, using fear and moralistic terms to talk about foods can lead to children being confused and fearful about eating, and can lead to restrictive eating.

Anna M. Lutz, nationally recognized family feeding specialist, agrees that our society's obsession with weight, fueled by fear-based public health messaging, has infiltrated parent culture in the past 10–15 years. Anna states, "We get the message that being a good parent means having a child with a certain-sized body. But parents are not in charge of their child's weight."

What are parents in charge of? Simply put, we believe a parent's job is to support their child(ren) in gaining skills, knowledge, confidence, peace, and independence. A focus on weight and dieting shows up in parenting in different ways. Diet culture influences how we talk about different foods and how we teach children about nutrition. Diet culture may influence what and how much we feed our children. If we work to parent in a diet-free way, we support our children to grow up practicing behaviors that support true health.

EATING IS SELF-CARE

Eating and self-care are just like other skills children learn over time. As parents, we support our children in learning to go to bed on their own, to develop study skills, and to drive a car. Taking care of oneself independently isn't something we need to expect our children to do when they are young. When you think about your child being grown up, and entering the world on their own, what skills or knowledge do you want them to have when it comes to eating and taking care of their body? Some examples may be:

- Feel relaxed and flexible around food.

- Know how to feed themselves in a way that is balanced, nourishing, and satisfying overall.

- Possess basic food preparation skills.

- Eat well and listen to their body.

- Have an appreciation for the wisdom and diversity of bodies.

None of these have to do with weight, as weight is not a behavior. Trying to control your weight or your child's weight interferes with a child developing these skills or behaviors that support true health.

BACK TO BASICS

We can get back to basics and parent in a diet-free way by providing appropriate structure regarding meals and snacks, and modeling healthy behaviors, rather than telling our children what or how much to eat. We encourage you to talk about food in neutral terms, rather than black-and-white categories of "good" and "bad." Separate talking about food and weight. Provide your children with first-hand experiences of a variety of foods. Allow children to have experiences of sometimes eating too much and sometimes too little, without judgment or commentary. Research shows that weight-inclusive and intuitive eating approaches have better physical and emotional health outcomes than approaches focusing on weight.[1, 2, 3]

STRUCTURE WITHOUT PRESSURE OR RESTRICTION

Diet culture in parenting shows up as parents dictating how much a child eats or the notion that a child needs to eat certain foods deemed healthy and/or totally avoid other foods. Diets use external rules that influence what and how much a person eats, rather than honoring internal cues. As parents, we want to support our children in listening to their internal cues and wisdom when it comes to interacting with the world, and this includes eating. Providing a supportive structure with food in the home supports children in doing just that.

Think about a child learning to go to bed. When our children are young, we provide them with a routine or a structure that helps them wind down at the end of the day. The routine may include a bath, a book, a song, and a kiss goodnight. This is structure. As they get older, you may start to slowly drop some of this structure, as they gain the skills to take care of themself and go to bed on their own. This is similar to providing a supportive structure in feeding.

Ellyn Satter is a well-known dietitian, family therapist, and feeding expert. She and her team have developed and researched the Satter Division of Responsibility in Feeding (sDOR), a way of feeding that supports children in growing up to have eating and self-care skills that foster health and well-being.[4] Satter's approach is the gold standard for preserving a child's relationship to their food and body image. Her approach is both weight-neutral and food-neutral. The goal of the sDOR approach is for young people to feel good about eating, trust themselves, and fuel their body in positive ways.

When thinking about supportive structure in your home, consider the timing of meals and snacks. sDOR explains that parents decide *when* it is time to eat and *what* is served. Provide regular meals and sit-down snacks, so that it is clear when it is time to eat and when it is not time to eat. As parents, we do the grocery shopping and understand the complex concepts of nutrition. Therefore, we provide the food items that are served at each meal and snack. Short-order cooking can prevent a child from expanding the foods they eat. Deciding when it is time to eat and what is served provides children with that supportive structure, so they can listen to their bodies and slowly expand their own eating skills.

It's important not only to be consistent in making food available in predictable ways but also to make sure the "what" to eat is varied to include all foods. The long-term goal is for our children to become adult eaters who eat a variety of foods and listen to their internal wisdom regarding how much they eat. For this to happen, they need to develop a peaceful relationship with all foods, not just those deemed "healthy." Structure is essential in supporting your child to listen to their body, eat new foods, and prioritize eating. Using dichotomous language regarding food, making foods good or bad, disconnects young people from their body's innate wisdom and causes them to overly respond to off-limits foods outside of the house.

Aim to provide three sit-down meals, and one to three sit-down snacks daily. Structure, in this case, is not restrictive; it provides guidance externally so that it can be internalized. Teens still need this structure as they are learning to be more independent with their food, the same way you might structure their social media use or give them a curfew. The structure gives them clarity and lets them know where they stand. They may experiment with it, but it gives them a place to anchor. Keep the structure in your mind in an overarching way. For example, you can decide if you want them to wait for dinner in an hour or fix them a snack; generally, it's important to assess this in real time. And in the beginning, it's trial and error. It will feel a bit ambiguous, but over time you will feel more confident guiding their food in a way that matches their developmental stage.

It's also important to not say too much about why you are making decisions about food. It can be as simple as, "It's not time to eat. Dinner will be in an hour." Otherwise, a justification may imply that you need one. Lengthy justifications allow teenagers to find loopholes and potentially use parental boundaries as a weapon.

SUPPORT YOUR CHILD IN KNOWING HOW MUCH

sDOR explains that the young person in your home is responsible for *whether* they eat the items offered, as well as *how much* they eat. Let's say you have served lasagna, salad, bread, and grapes. Once you have done this, take a deep breath and allow your child to decide if they are going to eat the items offered and how much. They may eat lots of lasagna and no salad. Or they may only try a bite or two of lasagna and eat grapes and bread.

So many factors go into how much a person eats at a particular time (including food preferences and familiarity with foods), and it's important to hold the structure so that your child can listen to their body, be exposed to different foods, and not be restricted. They may eat more or less of certain meals and snacks, but overall they will get the nutrition they need.

We suggest that your teen should have the autonomy to decide whether or not they want to eat. For example, say the teacher in their last period of school handed out a hearty snack in class, close to the time you regularly dole out an after-school snack. They may already be full, so instead of encouraging them to override their fullness, let them opt out. We don't want to disconnect them from their body's cues.

> Hunger and satiety cues will be suppressed in teens or children undergoing eating disorder treatment. This is due to chaotic dieting, weight loss in some cases, and malnutrition, which interfere with the metabolism. In these cases, it can take time for the body's natural hunger and fullness cues to be re-established. Often, to do this, parents will implement a regular feeding schedule, through which they take over all aspects of their child's food intake, meal planning, and even plating, until the eating disorder has receded sufficiently for the child to resume these activities on their own. This is known as Family-Based Treatment and is the first line of treatment for adolescents with eating disorders.

Teens are also in charge of their stopping place (with the exception of eating disorders as noted above). This can be the hardest for parents to bear witness to, and also one of the most important. It's important that they learn this one experientially. It can be difficult if you, as the parent, may be working on getting back to trusting yourself and strengthening your own competence in eating. The goal is for them to eat in full view of you. If you are micromanaging their slices of pizza, for example, you are increasing the likelihood that they may start to sneak pizza or overly respond to pizza outside of the home. Trust that their body knows how much it needs.

There's one exception to consider: if your child is claiming their fifth slice of pizza, and there will not be enough to go around, it's okay to manage the amount of food they take. This is more about good manners and making sure everyone has had their fair share, rather than concern about their weight. In other words, *pay attention to your intention*. When the intent is rooted in a weight concern, parents often think they can be innocuous about it, especially when kids are younger. As your child enters into their teen years, they will be on to you and realize, "They don't want me to have another slice of pizza, because they are worried I'm going to gain weight."

Lutz noted:

> Teens have the ability to know how much they need to eat, and when we interfere with that, as parents, we start to break down their natural ability. When we model that we trust our children to listen to their bodies, that they are in charge of their bodies, it also models consent.[5]

Who doesn't love a cookie exchange, where you bake large quantities of one cookie and then swap dozens, or half-dozens, with a group of friends and fellow bakers? This can be a fun way to have a variety of cookies in the house, without having to bake all of the variations yourself. This is also a type of setting in which you would want the structure with food, as the parent, to be flexible. If your child is present, they might feel embarrassed or restricted if they are allowed less access to the cookies than other guests. And you certainly don't need to worry about your child taking so many cookies that others won't have their share—there's a plethora of cookies!

But what if you saw them eating so many cookies they were likely to feel sick? It may be hard, but we encourage you to allow them to learn experientially from this experience. Eating in a way that does not honor their future self is a great opportunity to learn. Sometimes, we learn more from our perceived mistakes than we do when we are doing things perfectly. This kind of experiential learning in real time goes a lot further than any preventative measure a parent could take. We want to do our best to not get in our children's way; by learning first-hand what it's like to eat "too much" sometimes, and maybe other times eat "too little," teens—and adults—come to understand our body's needs and limits.

TOO STRICT, TOO LOOSE, JUST RIGHT

We have noticed, and research reveals, that parenting styles that are too strict with food (we call this externally imposed restriction) or too loose with food tend to backfire. Households with parents who externally impose restrictions are more likely to have kids that sneak food, hoard it, and overly respond to it when they have autonomy outside of the home. This is a risk factor for disordered eating and eating disorders. And as healthism and morality in food are on the rise, eating disorder professionals are seeing an uptick in these behaviors in their caseloads. (The term "healthism" was coined by Robert Crawford in the 1980s.[6] It refers to the achievement of well-being through lifestyle modifications. Healthism implies that an individual's health is a result of individual choices and behaviors, and ignores social determinants of health, such as a history of trauma, experiencing racism, not having access to safe housing, and inadequate access to nutritious food.)

Being too loose can manifest in numerous ways: teens being in charge of their meals/snacks, parents constantly short-order cooking, or non-existent family mealtimes. This gives teens too much "moving around room" with food. Another example of "too loose" would be allowing the young person in your home to experiment with fad diets. This sometimes sneaks under the radar, leaving parents feeling helpless and surprised—"We didn't notice it at first, it just seemed like they were eating 'healthier' and exercising more!" Dieting at any level has been termed the "most important predictor of eating disorders."[7, 8, 9, 10, 11]

Eating disorders have existed throughout history. However, eating disorders rates are increasing markedly.[12] There is data to indicate that during the era of public health campaigns to fight the "obesity epidemic," eating disorders rates have doubled. Between 2000 and 2006 there was a 3.5 percent worldwide eating disorder rate. From 2013 to 2018, the worldwide eating disorder rate was 7.8 percent. (These prevalence rates don't capture subclinical eating disorders or disordered eating, which are just as physically and emotionally harmful.) Well-intentioned public health campaigns have influenced medical care, parenting advice, and the media.

TEACHING CHILDREN ABOUT NUTRITION

In child development centers and schools, current education is based on what is developmentally appropriate, and educators match the content to the specific developmental stage of their students. *Except with nutrition.* Our culture's focus on weight and fears about food have hijacked developmentally appropriate ways to teach children about nutrition and food, and this also translates to the home. Fear-based nutrition education and developmentally inappropriate nutrition education can lead to children being preoccupied with food, being fearful of certain foods, and developing disordered eating, especially for those with risk factors of developing an eating disorder.

Most nutrition concepts require abstract thinking skills and cognitive abilities that are not developed until middle school. Young children may interpret nutrition concepts in black-and-white terms and may become fearful and restrictive of certain foods. In domains outside of food and body image, we don't hesitate to teach our children in ways that match their stage of cognitive development. Consider this: at a neighborhood watch meeting, police might share statistics revealing that most burglars come in through the backyard when breaking into a house. This is important information for homeowners. However, we wouldn't share that information with our children, who might feel frightened or, as a result, have trouble sleeping. Instead, we store it away as something helpful to know as the adult in the house. Adults can absorb information like this and factor it into our broader understanding of home security, a task that requires abstract thinking. Abstract thinking is required to fully understand nutrition and health concepts, and to integrate them in a helpful, practical way.

Given this, why do we share all the details of food, health, and bodies with young children? Simple; *fear of fat*. We believe that if we teach young children the concepts of nutrition, we will prevent children from being in large bodies. Not only is this false—bodies come in all shapes and sizes—it also causes harm. As long as our society has fatphobia, we will also have eating disorders. We suggest you hold on to specific nutrition information and the link between nutrition and health, and not share the details when kids are younger. A parent may want to explain to a child all of the health reasons why they need to eat more fruits and vegetables, or the link between certain foods and heart disease. But this information is abstract and complex for a young child. A young child or a more sensitive older child may become scared to eat the food they are taught will cause heart disease. Or they may feel confused and fearful when a parent feeds them something they were taught was "bad" for them.

Instead, it's developmentally appropriate to teach young children where foods come from, prepare and cook food together, and expose them to a variety of foods, through no-pressure taste tests and learning about the diversity of food of different cultures. Young children learn from interacting with their world and having hands-on experiences. Young children learn about food and nutrition best through the example set in the home—the food that is served, regular family meals, and witnessing family members taking the time to stop and eat.

As children get older, around middle school age (11–13/14 years old), they begin to develop more abstract thinking abilities. They begin to be able to understand the link between food and health in more abstract terms and utilize the information in a helpful way. This is a developmentally appropriate time to start teaching children about food groups, how to put together balanced meals and snacks, and cooking skills. As they gain abstract thinking skills, teens can be taught more about the nutrition of food. However, it remains important to talk with teens about food without any connection with weight and without moralistic terms like "good" or "bad." They can learn about food groups or putting together balanced snacks, without the moralistic commentary of diet culture. Nutrition can be taught without the mention of weight or body size.

EXPOSURE TO ALL FOODS

Naturally, parents provide the food in the household, but what if the food they bring in is *too* healthy? There are so many confusing and contradictory nutrition messages it's not surprising that many have lost their way with food as a culture. Eating only "healthy" food is not healthy. Our children need real-life experiences with all different kinds of foods, so they can navigate the food scene out in the world. We don't want to reduce food choices to nutrients only, leaving out important aspects of food such as socialization, pleasure, and fun. We encourage you to experiment with and enjoy all kinds of food and present them in a matter-of-fact way. "Snack today is chocolate chip cookies with milk" is presented as matter-of-factly as "apples with peanut butter." That way, we don't give the cookies special power that they don't have. Cookies are going to be a bit more of a "party in your mouth" than the apples, so glorifying them will make them even sweeter than they inherently are.

WHAT ABOUT DESSERT?

Keeping desserts off-limits, or putting requirements on them, only makes desserts more desired and sought after. Instead of restricting desserts, have them as a joyful part of your family's eating, in order to provide your teen with opportunities to interact with them, enjoy them, and develop a healthy relationship with all foods. Restricting desserts or other highly palatable foods has been shown to lead to sneak eating or eating more of these foods, including in the absence of hunger. The frequency with which you serve dessert is up to you. If your household is recovering from a history of *externally imposed restriction*, then you might want to serve dessert every night for a while, as the family works on repairing their relationship to dessert foods. Otherwise, some nights you might have it and other nights you might not. You can simply state, "We're having dessert tonight" (or not), but, again, don't say a whole lot about it.

Satter suggests that if a dessert is offered with a meal, parents should offer a child-sized portion; this is an exception to the child deciding how much. Satter's approach also notes that if a dessert food is served as a snack, the young person is in charge of their stopping place, which allows them to experience eating until they are satisfied. This approach provides the child with different opportunities to interact with and enjoy desserts, without rules of having to earn them or perform. Allow your child to eat "too much" dessert at a snack sometimes, or eat their cookie before eating their protein at a meal. These real, lived experiences help them learn first-hand.

Listen. We know it's tempting to micromanage the food your teen has eaten during the day without you, but we suggest acting the opposite of those urges. Instead of saying, "You said you had a sweet roll at the snack bar this morning at school, so we aren't having dessert tonight," *simply don't assess what they ate.* The body doesn't freak out the way diet culture does. ("Oh no! Batten the hatches! It's another sweet roll coming down!") Nope. The body uses enzymes to break food down into smaller molecules, during the digestive process anyway.

We often hear parents say, "You can't have your dessert if you don't eat your broccoli." We encourage parents to think about what their goal is with vegetables. If the goal is to get your child to eat more vegetables *today*, then that might work. If the goal is to zoom out and think, "Okay, I want an adult child who will eat vegetables and enjoy a variety of foods," then parents really need to back up and stick to that structure we talked about. *Pressure does not equate to a child eating more vegetables.* Forcing a child to eat their broccoli not only teaches them that broccoli may taste bad but also encourages them to ignore their bodies in order to get dessert.[13]

The best way to teach children about nutrition and to listen and honor their bodies is through modeling. If a teen sees their parent taking the time to stop and eat balanced meals, they learn this is an important part of self-care. Instead of dieting, model eating adequately and not using external rules to determine what and how much you eat. Young people can sniff out incongruences between what we do and say, so it won't be enough to omit diet talk, but still eat quinoa while the family is eating pizza. It is certainly understandable that you would have your own fear around weight and food, given the culture we are living in, but we encourage you to really lean into the exercises at the end of each chapter, so that you can integrate the material and develop your own deep understanding of non-diet approaches to food, as well as weight inclusivity and size diversity. As you integrate these concepts, you will be able to both model and discuss them with your teen.

DIET-FREE PARENTING SELF-ASSESSMENT

We've discussed how dieting and a focus on weight disrupt a child's ability to eat in response to their body's wisdom and can lead to disordered eating, eating disorders, depression, and more. We talked about ways you and your family can move away from diet culture and move toward a more connected way of eating. The following exercise can help you evaluate where you and your family are, so you can determine where you'd like to be.

If you are in a two-parent relationship and questioning whether your co-parent/partner has eating difficulties that they might be externally imposing on the young people in your home, score for them; alternatively, each parent can take their own assessment and discuss.

DIET-FREE PARENTING SELF-ASSESSMENT

	Always = 3	Sometimes = 2	Rarely = 1	Never = 0
1 I speak about food in moralistic terms and label them as "good" or "bad."	☐	☐	☐	☐
2 I do not trust myself with all foods in the house.	☐	☐	☐	☐
3 I have resistance to allowing my child to be in charge of their stopping place with food.	☐	☐	☐	☐
4 I worry that if I have foods I've deemed "unhealthy" in the house, that's all my kids would eat.	☐	☐	☐	☐
5 I'm concerned that if I leave it to my child to decide whether or not to eat the vegetables I provide at mealtimes, they will never eat them.	☐	☐	☐	☐
6 I comment negatively on others' appearance. (I make comments about my kids' appearance/weight, I make comments about my spouse/partner's weight, I make comments about others' weight.)	☐	☐	☐	☐
7 I make negative comments about my own body.	☐	☐	☐	☐
8 I do not model eating full meals and taking the time to stop and eat.	☐	☐	☐	☐
9 I am involved in helping to structure my teen's meals (3 meals + sit-down snacks).	☐	☐	☐	☐
10 I step in when I think my child has had too much to eat.	☐	☐	☐	☐
11 I fear that my child will gain too much weight.	☐	☐	☐	☐
12 I do not have self-trust around dessert foods in the house.	☐	☐	☐	☐
13 I put requirements on my teen to get dessert (only if they eat their veggies, clean their plate, have not had other sweets that day...).	☐	☐	☐	☐

TOTAL SCORE: _____

Tally your points. Lower scores reflect a more peaceful relationship with food. If your score is 19 or higher, we advise you to meet with an experienced, weight-inclusive, non-diet registered dietitian and/or therapist for guidance around your own relationship with food and body.

Chapter 6

The Hunger Meter

LEARNING OUR BODY'S LANGUAGE

What is your relationship to hunger? Are you someone who "eats for hunger to come" or are you one of those expert over-riders who regularly denies being hungry until you're Hungry Like the Wolf (#sorrynotsorry for the 1980s reference)? What about fullness? Dieting and eating with "discipline" interrupts the natural process of listening to our body, since the intellectual mind arbitrarily overrides the body's natural needs. Eating in response to your body's wisdom will guide you on what to choose, when to eat, and how much to have, which is essential to becoming a confident, intuitive eater.

Food can be comforting, and there is nothing wrong with that. Sometimes you might turn to food intentionally, as it can be soothing. You might be craving something other than food, but then find yourself reaching for food without hunger, which is a perfectly normal part of a peaceful relationship with food. At mealtimes, it might be challenging to decode whether you are physiologically hungry or experiencing other feelings instead. That's where the Hunger Meter—a tool that helps create awareness and cultivate curiosity between you and your food—can help. By taking a sacred pause and asking yourself where you are on the Hunger Meter, you can increase your awareness, which can allow you to make an informed decision about eating. This can be especially helpful if stress-related eating has become more frequent. The Hunger Meter is one of our most helpful tools for getting back to a more connected way of eating.

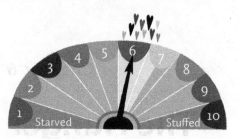

STARTING PLACES
Level 1

Usually at this level, you're ravenous. Andie, a 12-year-old, describes this stage: "A '1' is like I'm starving to death, feed me now, just give me anything and I swear I will eat it." You may feel dizzy or extremely cranky. Your brain, depleted of fuel, may cause you to feel as if it can't think clearly. You may feel weak and fatigued. It might be hard to focus on what you are doing. Remember the last time you skipped a meal because you had to hop on a call or something really important came up? Remember how suddenly and fiercely hungry you felt after things settled down? When here, you'll have difficulty stopping at "just enough." Eating in this zone of the meter can have a rapid, almost out-of-your-mind quality to it, so it's easy to miss a comfortable stopping place.

There can also be an obsessive quality that comes with this level. Let's say you reach Level 1 while you are finishing up a meeting. You can identify your hunger, but there is no food easily available. Your mind may think about food over and over again in an obsessive way. It will go something like this: "I'm hungry." Two minutes pass. "I wonder what I should make for lunch?" One minute passes. "Maybe I can run to the store and grab my favorite deli sandwich?" Thirty seconds pass. "No, that will take too long. I think I'll nuke the leftovers from last night's dinner." One minute passes. "I bet I could also find some salad to add to it." Meanwhile, you just missed the last ten minutes of whatever was happening in your meeting, because all you can think about is how to get your hands on some food. Extreme hunger can be very distracting.

When you're under-fueled and hungry, your blood sugar drops. This signals to the body to begin to break down muscle for fuel. Breaking down muscle gives the body some fuel, which may cause you to feel less hungry. But this is not the preferred way, of course—most of us want our muscles!

At this stage, you might over time begin to feel less hunger and think, "I'm not really hungry anymore." Um, yes, you are. You've just let your hunger go underground, and now you're momentarily getting a "second wind."

Level 2

At Level 2, you have slightly more control than at Level 1. You may not have as many physiological symptoms, such as dizziness or fatigue, and your brain may be a little sharper. But you are still very hungry. Your stomach may be rumbling loudly and you may be getting some weird looks from people nearby.

Similar to Level 1, you will also be at risk for overeating. The intensity of hunger may propel you to take more food than your body really needs, or eat so quickly that you bypass your brain's ability to recognize that it's full. (It takes the brain some time to catch up to the stomach and register that you are full—usually about 20 minutes.)

Food needs to be broken down or digested. This is a complex system, but the end goal is to take the important nutrients from your food and ship them over to the parts of your body that need them (calcium to your bones, for example). This pathway of complex signals and deliveries happens quickly, but not instantly. Thus, your brain doesn't know that you are full right away. This is why eating regularly and slowly is important, so that you don't overdo it when you're famished, and then end up stuffed and uncomfortable.

Level 3

Ahhh, now we're arriving at a manageable hunger. You feel calm and mindful about the decision to eat. You're not ravenous, but you may feel a little twinge in your stomach, a little emptiness telling you that your body wants food. You know it's been a while since you had your last meal, and you feel ready to find food so that your brain and body can perform at an optimum level. There is less drama here at Level 3. You're not obsessing about food, your brain is functioning well, and your body feels healthy. But it's time to eat, and you can calmly consider, "What do I want to eat?" To determine what it is you actually want to eat, tune in and decide from the inside what *taste*, *texture*, and *temperature* you'd like your food choice to be.

Discovering Your 3 Ts

The 3 Ts (taste, texture, and temperature) work best if your hunger is at a manageable place on the Hunger Meter. When you get the first inkling that you are hungry, tune in and decide from the inside what it is you'd like to eat this go-around.

- **Taste:** are you looking for something salty, like pretzels? Sweet, like chocolate? Or savory, like cheese and crackers?

- **Temperature:** do you want something cold and refreshing like watermelon? Or warm and soothing, such as soup?

- **Texture:** are you looking for something crunchy, like

chips? Chewy like dried fruit? Or soft, like yogurt or ice cream?

Level 4

This is the gray zone and harder to describe. You might not have many physical cues telling you that you are hungry, but you probably *could* eat. If lunch is at noon, and you have a break for a snack at 2 p.m., you might find that you are a 4 on the Hunger Meter around this time. You could eat, but you're not that hungry. At Level 4, you may also feel snacky. If something's really tempting, such as a banana and peanut butter, you might say yes, but you might also say no.

Level 5

You've probably just eaten and probably aren't physiologically hungry. At this point, your pull toward food is likely due to *something else*. What do I need right now? Emotions often signal a need. If you hang out with an emotion long enough, you might, for example, identify a feeling of boredom. Feeding boredom won't alleviate your original desire. Are you craving solitude or socialization? Does the idea of going for a hike tire you or inspire you? Do you crave more time with your family? Less time with your family (ha ha)? It's good to have a list of fun activities to do when you get into this zone that doesn't have anything to do with food (we call this foodless fulfillment).

EATING TO APPETITE

Your appetite may not be a morning person; not all of us are! To keep your body's metabolism on track, you should be diving into that initial meal within the first hour of getting up. It's important to keep your metabolism alert and operational by eating regularly throughout the day. Eating every 3–4 hours is a good way to teach yourself to feel hungry throughout the day, while preventing you from feeling ravenous later on.

For example, let's say you wake up at 7 a.m. Perhaps breakfast is at 7.30 a.m. Depending on what time you have lunch, you might need a snack mid-morning at 9.30, when your stomach starts rumbling. Aim for lunch by noon, snack at 3 p.m., dinner at 6, and an evening snack at 9. In an ideal world, teens would go to bed and wake at the same time each day for optimal sleep patterns. But should your teen sleep in, and you're up at 11 that morning, everything just gets shifted. Breakfast would be at 11, lunch at 2 p.m., snack at 4 or 5, dinner at 8, and snack at 10 or 11.

As you become more comfortable with this, you can eventually transition to eating in response to your body's hunger cues. When you get hungry will depend on when, what, and how much you last ate—which seems incredibly obvious, but if you're used to loitering mindlessly on the Hunger Meter all day, it may take considerable listening skills to learn to decode what your body is telling you.

STOPPING PLACES
Level 6
You can eat again when you get hungry, we promise; this is not your last chance! Your stomach feels happy and at peace; it's not overly stuffed and not looking for more. Your future self will totally dig that you were able to stop at just enough. Stopping at Level 6 leaves most people feeling energized after eating. In American culture, this feeling is most common at lunchtime.

Level 7
You've passed Level 6, and are feeling a little more anchored by your food. Fun fact: our taste buds lose interest much beyond this point. Just another cool thing the body does to let us know we're at a nice stopping place.

Level 8

You are on the path toward full. You might not like this feeling if "bow pose" is in your near future, but otherwise, no big deal. (Bow pose is a yoga pose where you lie face down on your mat, then bend your back into the shape of an archer's bow.)

Level 9

This is Thanksgiving Dinner full. You are uncomfortable here, and you're feeling as if you just want to crash on the couch and not do much. Although you're fueled, you're not feeling particularly energized. You ate past the point of energy, and you probably just want to nap.

Level 10

Time to unbutton! You're stuffed. It happens. No one loves feeling this way. Andie, age 12, describes this feeling as, "I'm so full I'll explode to 100%." At this point, there's not a whole lot to do here, other than breathe. This uncomfortable feeling will likely serve as a disincentive to finding your way back to a "10" anytime soon. Allow your body to do what it knows how to do—digest and process the food, which it will do. And don't stress. Feeling guilty and shameful doesn't make anything better. Some meals/days will be like this. Practicing the Hunger Meter will allow you to tune in and happily feel satisfied with food.

STOPPING AT JUST ENOUGH

Most people find stopping at just enough is the most difficult guideline for connected eating. Although food tastes yummy, once you start eating beyond satisfaction, your taste buds begin to become de-synthesized or toned down.

Stopping at just enough is complicated. Not only is it ideal to start at a 3 on the Hunger Meter so you can read your hunger, but you also have to feel satisfied emotionally and physically about your choice. If you're regularly eating for reasons other than hunger, you probably won't be satisfied by what you eat, and you may realize that you're filling another kind of need. It's like the game a Whack-a-Mole at the fair, where the mole (your emotion) pops up and you try clubbing it down with the hammer of food. In case you aren't familiar with this game, no matter how many times you whack those moles, they just keep popping up over and over again. Ultimately, you've gotta learn to love the moles and ask them what they need.

> When you feel a pull toward food, create space between you and the food to see where you are on the Hunger Meter.

Hunger Meter: From Ravenous to Just Right

1 = Ravenous, dizzy, cranky, can't think clearly, low blood sugar

2 = Very hungry, rumbling stomach

3 = Manageable hunger, a happy place where you want to arrive at mealtime, calm and mindful about eating

4 = You could eat, but you're not that hungry; snacky

5 = You've probably just eaten, and aren't hungry

6 = The dreamy stopping place; your stomach feels happy and at peace, but it's not overly stuffed

7 = Your taste buds lose interest much beyond this point

8 =   You are on the path toward full and feel anchored
        by your food

9 =   Thanksgiving Day stuffed

10 = Time to pull on the PJ pants

Ultimately, the key is to match your fuel to your hunger level. For example, if you are a 4, you might need a small snack, such as fruit with a small handful of nuts. If you are a 1 on the Hunger Meter—that is, basically starving—you probably need a full meal. Just an apple will not do. As your blood sugar comes back to normal, ask yourself, "Why was I so hungry? Did I miss something that day? Was my lunch not filling enough?"

Whether it's time for a meal or snack, we recommend eating when arriving at a manageable hunger, or a 3 on the Hunger Meter—a place that is somewhere between not too hungry and not too full. You feel calm and mindful about the decision to eat. You're not ravenous, but you may feel a little twinge in your stomach, a little emptiness telling you that your body wants food. It's been a few hours since you had your last meal, and you feel ready to find food so your brain and body can perform at an optimum level.

Factors including what taste, texture, and temperature of food you are in the mood for—sweet, smooth, creamy, crunchy, hot, or warm—can help you figure out what to eat. If you pause and identify that you are on the fullness end of the Hunger Meter—say an 8, 9, or 10—you might be curious why you're reaching for chips. If you are a 9 on the Hunger Meter—meaning you are pretty full—you're likely not physiologically hungry at all.

When feeling a pull toward food at an 8 to 10, the focus is not so much on whether or not you end up eating the food or not, but instead should be on strengthening your ability to create space and cultivate curiosity about why you're seeking out food if you're not hungry. Sometimes, a simple question and answer with yourself can help you to see what's really going on. For example, if you are not hungry for food, try asking yourself, "What am I really hungry for?" Maybe it's a nap you really want, or maybe you just need a morning to yourself, with no Zoom meetings or appointments.

Then again, you may just want cookies, even if you are full. And that's okay! You can certainly eat dessert without hunger, and in that case, it may be fulfilling a need for pleasure. But if this happens chronically or habitually, in a way that makes you uncomfortable, you might want to ask yourself, "If it wasn't about the cookie, what would it be about?" If you determine that eating the cookies grounds you at the end of a long day, maybe switch it up a bit and try yoga or writing in your journal. Think of foodless fulfillment as a way to increase your pleasant activities—these pursuits can fill you up from the inside in a way that food without hunger cannot.

ALL FOODS AND OCCASIONS FIT

Ultimately, it's important to remember that all foods fit as part of a healthy diet, and it's not so much about what or how much you choose to eat or not eat—rather, the journey is about becoming more self-aware. Awareness brings choices. Only you can know what you'd like your stopping place to be; it's very personal. At your favorite restaurant, for example, you may wish to feel a bit more anchored by your food and stop at an 8, whereas stopping at a 6 at lunch on a workday may help you feel more energized. It's not about judging your choices. Diet culture likes to demonize choices, but we encourage you to adopt an "all foods fit" mentality. You might have ice cream one night and strawberries the next night, and both work!

Do you know when you're hungry? How about when you've

had "just enough" at a meal? Understanding hunger and fullness cues are skills that are innate to all of us, but they might require a little practice. Eating in response to your body's wisdom will guide you on what to choose, when to eat, and how much to have, which is all anyone needs to be a confident, intuitive eater.

Chapter 7

Ingredients for Building a Peaceful Relationship with Food

There are several ingredients required for helping your family build a healthy relationship with food. This will help not only with building meals that everyone enjoys but will make mealtimes more pleasant. This chapter is loaded with information; use what speaks to you and reject the rest. Food choices are expansive and can be highly personal. The panorama of food can be influenced by individual preferences, culture, seasonality, global and regional trends, cravings, peer influences, food availability, and food access (grocery stores, farmer's markets, access to transportation, bike paths or walkways to access locations).

Food is so much more than protein, starch, and vitamins and minerals, yet many people struggle to really have fun with food. We also have different foods for different situations, ages/stages, and occasions. Think of the foods we might eat for socialization (birthday parties) and for cultural reasons (like a family reunion). Food is meant to add joy, fun, and pleasure. It is a central ingredient in socialization, bringing families, friends, and loved ones together for holidays, special events, celebrations, sporting events, and concerts.

Food culture can be considered in multiple ways. We have community culture, which is often related to a dominant group within a population. For example, the United States is inextricably linked to the image of the American burger. French culture is forever known for its croissants and pastries. Indian food is usually associated with spicy cuisine, and Caribbean food can sometimes be limited by the idea that it is "island food" or "tropical," despite the fact that there are influences and shared recipes with many communities from around the world. Despite these cultural associations, the reality is that not everyone eats similarly to the mainstream community in which they live and work.

We often see teens attempt to reject the foods that are native to their family—whether that be to assert independence, assimilate with peers, or rebel, or simply as a way of fitting into the dominant culture. Diet and health views quickly find their way into this rejection, with many kids saying their parents' food is too "heavy" and "not healthy," which is particularly interesting as we see this sentiment repeated across cultures and cuisines. This dynamic can be hurtful for parents and grandparents who want to impart their traditions through food. It is our view that all foods, cuisines, and plates can be part of a well-balanced diet that provides not only all of the nutrition necessary to support growth and development but also a sense of family, belonging, and values.

Privileged eating in its simplest form is being able to eat what you want, when you want, how you want, and without concern for accessibility or affordability. As we examine food beliefs and navigate ways to stay nourished, it is vital that we consider the privilege of being able to make food choices. However, as we explore expansive ways to eat and live, we must also discuss the ways in which many adults and children suffer food insecurity. While it may be tempting to think that this happens in other parts of the world, the reality is that many individuals in local communities struggle with gaining and maintaining sufficient or consistent access to food, or the ability to afford it.

Below are some ideas for putting meals together for your teen and family, both at home or on the go, in the context of food access and in an effort to support the goals of developing a peaceful relationship with food now and in the future. As you consider how you want to nourish your family and consider what foods you want to eat, we encourage you to pick widely, to enjoy the gifts that choice allows you, and to consider supporting organizations that serve underserved communities. If for no other reason than the fact that when someone is hungry there is *no* "evil food" and *no* "junk food," we ask you to rethink and abandon food stigma and mainstream cultural ideas of what constitutes "good" and "bad" food, and simply eat. We encourage you to embrace food diversity and fully reject diet culture, as it can often lead to narrow ideas of acceptable food, and create an extreme relationship of what is and is not allowed. By welcoming food diversity, we can create space to introduce varied foods and cultures into our own households.

MAKE FOOD EQUAL IN AVAILABILITY

Let's say you're in a time crunch and you run into the house to grab a snack. Both a bag of Halloween candy and the "makings" for a sandwich are readily available. The easier choice is the candy, since the sandwich isn't made. The candy tastes great but will not give you sustained energy. You're stuck because you don't have the time (or maybe the desire) to make a sandwich, even though you would have been more satisfied with one. This example highlights the importance of making foods not only equal in morality but also equal in availability. The point isn't that candy is bad or a sandwich is good, but that without proper planning you might gulp down whatever is quickest, instead of what your body actually needs. The highest goal is to have a fridge full of foods you know your body does really well with, but also to feel calm and grounded when you'd like candy (not frantic or impulsive, but a calm 3–4 on the Hunger Meter). Sandwiches and candy are different, but they all have value.

Some may worry that getting specific groceries days ahead will make planning difficult, given that we don't know what we are going to crave later today, let alone three days from now. Don't worry about buying food in advance without knowing "the plan" for the week. When possible, grab staples to keep around that you know you and your family enjoy. Keeping some shelf-stable foods around—rice, pasta, beans, frozen foods—plus adding in some proteins as well as fruits and vegetables (frozen/canned are okay, too!) enables us to assemble variations of favorites with little fanfare. If you can plan ahead, then do so. Sometimes this helps to manage time, last-minute stress about what to cook, and your own hunger, as well as your child's hunger. Pause and get a sense of what works for you and your family. Do you prefer to improvise in the kitchen, or carefully plan out a week's worth of meals? There's no right answer, but there *is* likely an easier choice for your household.

Making food equal in availability requires preparation. This may mean having a stash of previously agreed-upon on-the-go foods in your teen's backpack, locker, or car. This is especially important if they tend to override their hunger because they choose to wait until they get home. Some kids (and adults) have a lack of interoceptive awareness (a fancy phrase for the ability to respond to internal signals, such as knowing when you should eat or go to the bathroom). Instead, those teens might need to eat more mechanically, by the clock rather than relying on their body's innate wisdom. Also, keep in mind that certain medications, stressful experiences, sleep deprivation, and other circumstances can stimulate or suppress hunger and satiety cues. The same can be true for certain medical conditions, including eating disorders, thyroid and other endocrine disorders, gastrointestinal disorders, or inflammatory disease, to name a few. In these and other circumstances, specific nutritional plans will be needed, in order to make sure that an individual is appropriately nourished.

VARIETY IS THE...

We encourage variety in meal planning when possible and within reason. During the early months of the COVID-19 pandemic, many families were forced to adapt on the fly when stores ran out of food. This was hard for those used to only buying specific items. Rigidity around food intake can make it challenging for kids to eat when at friends' houses, traveling, or when heading off to college. The more we practice flexibility, the easier it will be for kids to navigate a variety of new circumstances. Kids who eat the same thing over and over again at lunch, for example, are also more likely to throw it away or skip part of it. This inevitably leads to ravenous hunger by mid-afternoon. Changing it up at meals and introducing new and novel foods can make eating seem more appealing, or even exciting. However, for some who have certain developmental or medical needs and are prone to more narrow food choices where repetition is more comforting, adding variety in diets can be more challenging.

Those who have children with a limited range of foods would benefit from "food cycling." Parents can literally cycle through the foods, even if limited, that their child does eat. Changing cereals, serving different shaped pastas, or using different breads can create a new experience for a child with limited eating options. This can be beneficial in getting kids to expand out of their comfort zone, and can eventually be a gateway to more culinary adventures in the future. Food flexibility has nutritional benefits, as well. Variety helps us take in different nutrients each day without having to think too much about it. For example, if you just eat bananas, you might miss out on the Vitamin C found in an orange. Similarly, if you only eat chicken and turkey each day, you might miss out on the iron found in red meat.

As you model eating an array of different foods, your child may also be more inclined to experiment. Parents can increase the variety in their child's diet by rotating different types of fruits and vegetables consumed, and mixing up the meals served for breakfast, lunch, and dinner. Shopping in different supermarkets can help create a different rotation of snacks. We also recommended buying different brands, just to keep kids flexible with similar but slightly modified flavor profiles. New recipes, pot luck dinners, Pinterest recipes, farmers' markets, or even just bringing your kids with you when you shop can help to keep the food varied in your home. As we mentioned, we understand that balancing consistency and variety can be challenging. And we get it: there are only so many things that you can do or so many recipes you can mix up. The messages here are not to add more to your plate (no pun intended), but it's to introduce and discuss some ways in which parents can promote food curiosity and avoid restrictive food behaviors.

ALL TOGETHER NOW

Family meals are an opportunity for family time that allows for household members to come together, leave behind the day, catch up with one another, and ideally recharge as well as reconnect. Research has shown that family mealtime is positively associated with teen academic performance, improved mental health, and even self-esteem.[1, 2, 3] Eating meals together can also help with eating disorder prevention, since parents can see what's on their child's plate and intervene or access help if necessary. Therefore, eating together can help with emotional, social, and physical health. Talk about bang for your buck!

Keep mealtime conversation light, fun, and stress-free. Allow the table to be a place where kids will want to be with others. Leave stressful conversations at the door and away from the table. If conversation stalls, you may wish to play a fun game like "Would You Rather?" Your family can ponder if they would rather be able to fly or be invisible, or rather speak every language in the world or play every musical instrument?[4] Consider simple conversation prompts (current events or what good things happened today) or other games (more available on The Family Dinner Project website). Music also helps set a vibe; let family members take turns DJ-ing shared meals. Families might also want to establish a set of table guidelines to honor the meal further, such as no screen use at the table, no interrupting each other, reciting "highs and lows of the day," and/or staying at the table until everyone is finished.

SCREEN-FREE EATING

A new normal has developed in the age of tech and has further developed since 2020: kids and parents are eating while logging on remotely from their computer. For some, virtual meetings or school have cut out commute times, allowing a little more bandwidth for having sit-down meals. However, in more cases than not, many may not be eating at all, or may be delaying mealtimes until online activities are done. Longer hours at the computer are shifting the ways in which people experience eating a meal, as well as feelings of satiety.[5] We are seeing an increase in mindless, distracted eating that has caused a disconnect to tasting, chewing, and even swallowing food. Think about the last time you ate at your desk while completing work. Do you remember tasting your food? Do you remember what you ate? Did you feel full or satisfied after your meal?

Screen time is here to stay. We need to be intentional about not being on electronics while eating. As we repeatedly practice and reinforce these behaviors, they become habitual. One definition of habit is something you start doing before you realize you are doing it. If this is the case when it comes to technology in your home, create a designated device space, AKA "the phone basket," where tech lives during family meals. Write "Be with the people who are *here*" on a Post-it, as a reminder to put away tech as you sit and connect with your loved ones. A 2020 study conducted in Greece found that adolescents who ate a meal or snack while on screens were less likely to eat with their families and more likely to miss breakfast.[6] In another study, researchers found that the mere presence of a cell phone negatively impacted the perception of closeness and connection and even conversation quality.[7] Take a break from screens to eat and engage with the other rich aspects of your life.

HAVE A SEAT

Why do kids love to stand and eat? And why do they also love to eat right out of the pantry? Some of this is normal and casual behavior for teens. Ideally, you'd want to encourage them to eat in a way they'd ask their friend to join them. You wouldn't think of inviting a friend over for dinner and standing with them in the pantry, would you?

Part of getting back to basics means asking teens to plate their food and eat sitting down. This brings with it secondary benefits, such as helping to make sure the meal is adequate and balanced. Sitting down and eating might help the person eating to slooooow down the pace. When we're eating on the go, we are less likely to notice what we're eating, its flavor or texture, and we may not fully register how fast we are eating. Plus, did you know that the anticipation of the meal actually helps to start the digestive process, by secreting enzymes necessary for digestion?

PUTTING IT ALL TOGETHER (NUTRITION 101)

All teens have a high energy requirement, given they are still growing and developing. Requirements are even higher for athletes, who tend to expend even more energy; this makes eating regularly especially important. This usually translates to three meals and two to three snacks per day.

Naturally, we recommend balanced meals, which feature a variety of food groups (starch, protein, vegetables/fruit, dairy, and fats), plus hearty snacks. This will provide satiety, while also providing the nutrients that everyone needs to thrive academically and athletically. A balanced nutrition plan not only fuels muscles but also powers the brain. This is fundamental for focus and being able to participate in chosen activities and sports at peak performance levels. Ingesting proteins and carbohydrates in combination—cheese and crackers together, for example—can slow down digestion and keep blood sugar levels more steady over time. This will also help with feeling full for a longer period of time. Alternatively, having something that is not as dense (perhaps just crackers) may not provide enough physical staying power.

Balanced meals ideally include the following:

Protein

Protein will help keep your teen full throughout the day and is important for muscle growth and repair, and synthesizing important enzymes that help your body work. It also plays a role in nail and hair growth! The American diet typically far exceeds the body's requirements for protein. Athletes do require more protein, but this is usually easy to accomplish. Those more at risk for having a low-protein diet are vegetarians, vegans, limited eaters, those with food allergies or dietary restrictions, or gastrointestinal disorders.

Parents often worry that their teen is not getting enough protein. It is fairly easy to meet these requirements for all teens, including those that may be vegetarian or vegan, by including a protein source at each meal. Adding vegan meatballs or soy crumbles to a tomato sauce are great ways to boost the protein content of a pasta dish. The vegan/vegetarian diet may be complicated for newbies and first-timers, due to a lack of familiarity and practice. We suggest consulting with a registered dietitian for questions and guidance.

Common sources of protein include chicken, turkey, tuna, steak, burgers, lamb, pork, ham, nut butters, eggs, hummus, cheese, yogurt, milk, tofu and soy (soy crumbles and other plant-based protein), beans and legumes (black beans, kidney beans, chickpeas, edamame, lentils, to name a few), seitan (wheat gluten, a vegetarian protein), and tempeh (vegetarian protein made from fermented soy proteins).

The following are key nutrients about which vegans/vegetarians should be aware:

- **Calories.** A great goal would be for plates to contain all five food groups (grains, proteins, fruits/vegetables, fats, and a dairy/dairy alternative source) and be full to ensure the meal is sufficient.

- **Protein.** Add a plant-based protein source at each meal to ensure protein intake is sufficient.

- **Vitamin B12.** Helps with the functioning of the

nervous system, DNA production, and red blood cell production. This vitamin is virtually absent in the vegan diet and needs to be consumed in fortified foods or taken via supplement. Sources include fortified cereals, nutritional yeast, and non-dairy milks.

- **Vitamin D.** Made in our bodies from sunlight, Vitamin D helps support bones, cell growth, and immune function. Mushrooms can be a source of Vitamin D if they are exposed to UVB radiation before consumption. Additional sources include dairy foods and milk, non-dairy milks, cereals, and margarines.

- **Calcium.** Helpful for building strong bones and teeth, muscle contractions, nerve transmissions, and blood pressure regulation. Sources include dairy from cow's milk, yogurt, kefir, and cottage cheese, or for vegans, non-dairy milk, tofu, soybeans, or "low-oxalate greens," including dark leafy greens, broccoli, bok choy, Chinese greens, kale, Napa cabbage, or turnip greens. Low-oxalate greens are a good source of calcium and are well-absorbed. But greens that are high in oxalates, such as spinach, are too high in oxalates, making the calcium largely unavailable to the body.

- **Iron.** Iron supports physical growth, brain development, energy, the immune system, and more. Plant sources of iron need to be paired with Vitamin C in order to maximize absorption. Plant-based iron sources include beans, raisins, black strap molasses, bars, cereals, and dark chocolate.

- **Omega 3 fats.** These must be obtained from the diet, and they help with cell membranes, hormones, clotting, and inflammation. Fatty fish such as salmon or tuna are the best dietary source of Omega 3 fatty acids. Vegetarian sources include eggs fortified with Omega 3s, chia seeds, flaxseed, walnuts; some might require a microalgae supplement.

We recommend consulting a non-diet registered dietitian for a comprehensive assessment. This is especially important for ensuring that growing adolescents are achieving their nutritional requirements.

Carbohydrates

Carbohydrates are the primary fuel source for your brain, heart, and muscles, and an important energy source, usually making up about 50 percent of one's diet. Parents often view carbs as a food group to reduce, or cut out entirely, due to concerns over weight, diabetes, or excess calories. Low-carb diets are glamorized and are often accompanied by quick weight loss, which is largely water lost when glycogen is depleted. It's easy to create a caloric deficit if you cut out 50 percent of your diet! But there's nothing magical here. That same caloric deficit could be created by reducing anything. And just like all diets, the results tend to be unsustainable in the long term and leave people feeling fatigued and craving the very foods they cut out.

Jake is a 16-year-old football player looking to bulk up. His parents noticed he started eating a lot of chicken, eggs, and steak, and drinking a lot of milk. He also wanted to add a protein supplement to his diet. Adding more protein may not be the answer, as many athletes are already exceeding protein recommendations. Instead, it may be helpful for him to add carbohydrates, larger meals, and additional snacks—consistently, to help him with his goal of bulking. A high-protein diet can make a person feel full, making it more difficult to stay on track with meals and snacks. If someone chooses to use a protein supplement, we recommend that the supplement be NSF (National Sanitation Foundation) certified[8] or third-party tested—meaning it's been tested to make sure that the supplement contains the ingredients listed on the label, are not contaminated (heavy metals, herbicides, pesticides), and do not contain banned substances.[9, 10] Also, check in with a non-diet dietitian or doctor to assess if this is something you actually need.

Caloric restriction, or dieting, can backfire. To top it off, as you have read throughout this book, dieting is the biggest predictor for the development of eating disorders. Avoiding foods and food categories polarizes foods for your children and may scare them about different foods and food groups. Why should they eat pasta, rice, and bread, if you don't? Your child is still growing and has high nutritional requirements during adolescence. We have found that those who intentionally restrict carbohydrates, such as rice and pasta, are more likely to binge on carbohydrate-rich foods later on.

SUGAR SUGAR

Yes, sugar is a carbohydrate. And no, sugar is not "poison." From parents to pediatricians to fitness bloggers, it seems everyone wants to comment on how much sugar we should or *shouldn't* be eating. Often, parents don't want sweets in the house because of their own self-trust issues around these foods. We encourage you to repair your relationship with sugar (if needed), rather than quitting sugar entirely.

Restricting sugar leads to confusion about how to engage with foods that contain sugar. Intentionally building self-trust around sweets outside of the house may be a necessary first step, before some people feel comfortable bringing them into the house. For example, go out and order a scoop or two of your favorite ice cream, and actually give yourself permission to eat it with pleasure. Creating these opportunities builds a sense of self-mastery, making it easier to bring a gallon of ice cream into the house. "All foods fits" is an ideal paradigm for a harmonious household.

Restoring Your Relationship with Sugar

If you find yourself craving sweet foods, take a beat and explore your feelings further. Ask yourself the following questions:

- Do you give yourself permission to eat sweets, or do you experience other (negative) feelings when you have them?

- Do you notice sweet cravings when you are very hungry or have skipped a meal? (This is common— and amazing. The body craves sweets when hungry because sugar is the quickest source of energy.)

- Do you find yourself eating more of one type of food when you are bored?

- Do you find yourself habitually seeking certain foods for pleasure or comfort? If so, it may indicate you need to increase your pleasant activities, outside of the arena of food and eating.

- The foods you crave most when you're not hungry can be telling. If it's sweets you crave, perhaps adding more of these foods on a more regular basis could help temper these cravings.

Sugar is a source of energy and it makes food tasty, sweeter, and usually more pleasurable. Foods with sugar are digested by the body into glucose molecules, and then used and stored as necessary. Our body's pancreas, when working, can secrete insulin to metabolize sugar like any other food particle that comes into the body. Sugar can be digested quickly, giving people quick access to fuel, whereas a sweet potato, for example, would take longer to digest. Much has been written about the differences here, but ultimately we are of the mindset that variety is the spice of life. We don't feel it's realistic or wise, let alone necessary, to mandate an avoidance of sugar. We recommend that sugary foods can be just another part of the diet that gets rotated or cycled through.

Sources of carbohydrates include oatmeal, cereals, bread (sour dough, whole grain, for example), potatoes (sweet potato and white potato), rice (white and brown), pasta, quinoa, couscous, and many snack foods such as cookies, chips, crackers, baked goods. Examples of whole grains include cereals, whole-grain crackers, or whole-grain breads. Whole-grain foods contain fiber, which can help with gastrointestinal health, and has been linked with improving heart health and helping with other health issues.

Fruit/vegetables

Add "color" to meals by adding fruits, vegetables, or both. A diet that is rich in fruits and vegetables can prevent constipation (sufficient water and other fluid intake is also vital for gastro-intestinal health and preventing constipation) and help with immune system health. Fruits and vegetables help athletes to recover after a long workout, minimize soreness, and help to reduce inflammation.

Some parents like microwaving veggies and serving them right out of the bag. There is nothing wrong with frozen vegetables and fruits (studies show they are nutritionally comparable), but you may need to "fun them up" to make them more appealing. Additions including butter, olive oil, dipping sauces (Ranch dressing, hummus, or guacamole) can increase flavor. Seasonings including salt, pepper, cheeses, Tajín® (a Mexican chili-lime seasoning, also great on mangos, cucumbers, and jicama!) are fun additions to fruits and vegetables. Keep exploring ways to prepare vegetables. Roasting them in the oven is pretty easy and tends to be a crowd-pleaser for broccoli, cauliflower, and Brussels sprouts.

When my family immigrated to the U.S., we traveled about 45 minutes each way to the ethnic grocery store to buy the spices and vegetables that weren't available elsewhere at the time. Spice mixes and other whole spices like cardamom are on a surprising number of grocery shelves now, but they didn't use to be. As my family lived in a major metropolitan city, we had access to specialty stores, but friends in more remote areas didn't have the same access and modified their food choices to accommodate what was available in local communities.

As I learned about and was increasingly exposed to local and regional "American" food, I developed an enduring love of milkshakes and nachos and so much more. However, it took a while for me to fully embrace and celebrate my food heritage. The inconvenience of getting Indian staples made them seem exotic and unnecessary, even to me, too. Well, that is until my mom made some of my favorites—mattar paneer (a traditional homemade cheese with peas in a spicy tomato curry) or rajma chawal (North Indian version of beans and rice).

I hesitated to take lunches to school, and I distinctly remember agreeing with a school friend when he asked if I was eating pork chops. I didn't know how to explain that what I was having was a tikki—a pan-fried, spiced potato and vegetable cutlet. This kid didn't have any ill intentions and was asking a question based on what was most familiar to him. In retrospect, I wish I had explained what I was eating, but to be perfectly honest, I was afraid. I was afraid of being made fun of for being different. Over time, off-hand mainstream jokes about Indian cuisine, how it will give you the runs, or comments like, "Geez, that's a strong smell" made me self-conscious, sometimes defensive, and even avoidant (not wanting to take friends to Indian restaurants).

Even as a young adult in medical school, during one instance of playful classmate banter, a friend called me "curry-slinger." In the moment, I laughed awkwardly, mainly because I didn't know what to say, but I was actually hurt by the comment. He didn't know that, and I didn't tell him. We remained friends, and he is a good person who I know didn't mean to be hurtful. However, stereotypes associated with food and the cultures that they come from can narrow perceptions of who people are. Through increased access to diverse foods, as well as a willingness to talk to people about their cultural food experiences, we can broaden our view of food possibilities. We can connect with others about what may be meaningful for them, and connect to their traditions. By the way, this doesn't have to be global cuisine. We can have preconceived notions and stereotypes about regional cuisine within our own nations and communities as well. Undoing these is just as important.

—*Shelley*

Fats

A fat source is recommended at each meal. This could be avocado, hummus, mayo, dressing, a dipping sauce, nuts, or a snack containing fats, such as a cookie or chocolate. Fats are good for the brain and body, and are needed to make important hormones like estrogen and testosterone, both of which help build strong bones. While estrogen and progesterone are present in males and females, in females specifically estrogen supports reproductive health, bone health, and even brain health, as well as other vital processes. Testosterone helps with vital functions and is particularly important for muscle mass and even strength in males and females.

People think fats can make you fat or that certain foods are "fattening." Neither is true, and this language perpetuates fear of fat, which is harmful to everyone, especially those living in larger bodies. Plus, it's scientifically inaccurate. One food does not have the power to cause weight gain. People think that dietary fats are the same as body fat, but they are not related at all. Fat makes food taste good, and makes food more fun and pleasurable. This makes us feel more satisfied and, in turn, we are likely to stop eating sooner. Like proteins, fats help to keep us feeling full throughout the day.

Dairy

Consider adding a dairy source, such as milk, chocolate milk, yogurt, kefir (probiotic smoothie), or cottage cheese. Greens including kale and spinach also contain calcium; however, they contain oxalates, making them less absorbable. Those who are lactose intolerant can choose lactose-free milks or use lactase enzymes before consuming dairy. Pea protein milk (Ripple Milk), fortified flax milk with protein (Good Karma), and soy milk all contain protein and calcium.

Calcium builds strong bones. Teens need 3–4 servings of dairy (or a dairy alternative source) per day. Optimizing bone density into your mid-20s, when "peak bone density" is achieved, will support lifelong bone health. That's why it's important for teens to have a lot of calcium during this unique window of opportunity.

Vitamin D is necessary for the absorption of calcium. Besides bone health, Vitamin D helps with injury repair, inflammation, growth, immune function, and metabolism.[11, 12, 13] Because of its role in immunity, Vitamin D deficiency received a lot of attention during the COVID-19 pandemic; low Vitamin D levels were associated with a worse response to Covid[14] and increased likelihood of death.[15] Supplementation with Vitamin D resulted in fewer respiratory infections[16] and is relatively cheap to accomplish. Before supplementing, find out where your/your teen's Vitamin D levels are (as assessed via bloodwork by checking 25-hydroxyvitamin D level).

Chapter 8

Diet-free Meal Prep for the Family

At this particular stage of life, your teen's meal prep skills might include using the toaster, a frying pan, and heck, they might even be able to wash a dish or actually *put it in the dishwasher*. We see some kids who are highly motivated to prepare and even shop for their food. Some turn to social media and platforms such as Instagram or Pinterest and enjoy the process of exploring and experimenting. Others, frankly, couldn't care less. This applies to adults, too! Whether they feel the Joy of Cooking or prefer the Joy of Not Cooking, convenience, cost, availability, mood, parental influence, and habit are all factors that influence adolescent eating patterns. Parents can help their kids by making foods readily available and easy to access.[1] Ellyn Satter says, "Despite acting like it doesn't matter, your adolescent continues to depend on you to maintain the structure of family meals. They will participate in family meals when you make meals a priority, keep mealtimes pleasant, and use mealtimes for connecting."[2]

NOW YOU'RE COOKING

Meals vary by culture and within families, and are highly personal. Without getting to speak one on one to each of you, any lists of meal ideas we might generate are likely to fall short of being able to address your unique food preferences, cooking skills, financial requirements, and needs. Below we have shared ideas for breakfast, lunch, dinner, and snacks, but, of course, we know these ideas won't entirely fit all readers. We hope instead that these lists will encourage and inspire you to brainstorm ideas that might work for your household.

BREAKFAST

Begin the day with a balanced breakfast, with all the food groups present. Kids often miss breakfast, but there is evidence to suggest that kids who eat breakfast have better memories, test grades, and school attendance. They also have greater focus, energy, and more nutrient-rich diets than those who skip breakfast.[3] This makes sense because breakfast-skippers are more likely to overeat later on, on unplanned foods, because they got too low on the Hunger Meter. We often describe metabolism to a teen as a fire you will want to keep well stoked throughout the day.

Breakfast ideas:

- oatmeal with almonds and strawberries, glass of milk*

- egg sandwich (egg, cheese), with your favorite fruit on the side

- gallo pinto (rice and beans), eggs, toast, plantains, glass of milk

- toast/hummus, tempeh slices, fruit, dairy-free milk

- Greek yogurt, granola, blueberries, nuts (parfait)

- bread, butter, ham/cheese, melon

- cereal and milk, banana slices, with sausage/turkey sausage on the side

- peanut butter on toast with banana slices, glass of milk

- pancakes with strawberries and butter, a smoothie.

* Can be made vegan with dairy-free milk such as soy milk, pea protein milk, or fortified flax milk with protein.

Some options found more commonly in East Indian households include parathas (flatbreads stuffed with various veggies, eggs, or meat), cheela (lentil or gram flour savory pancakes) served with cilantro-and-mint chutney or another dense chutney, idli (steamed rice and lentil cakes) in combo with a coconut chutney, ghee (clarified butter), and/or podi (dry condiment powder made from lentils or nuts, seeds, and spices), upma (savory cream of wheat cooked with nuts and vegetables) traditionally served with a chutney. The list is endless and can change based on regional modifications. Use the recipes that you and your family are familiar with to make hearty and satisfying meals.

What are some foods that are served in your household at this time of day?

LUNCH

You may be in charge of packing your teen's lunch for school. This is an important job because you have to think and prep ahead of schedule. Discuss with your teen what foods they want. Here, variety is important as our teens often complain about getting the "same thing every day." That said, some request the same thing every day, too! Changing up small things here, even for those with a limited range of preferences can be done by changing the fruits or vegetables, snacks, or switching the kinds of bread you are using. Sometimes we see parents sending a small thermos for their 16-year-old growing teen, and we ask them to switch that out to a bigger one if possible to add more food. Teens are becoming self-conscious and we know they can be particular. Their feedback is important. They may not want anything too loud (crunchy—depending on where they are eating it, perhaps in class for some), too smelly (tuna), or anything that gets mushy in their backpack (bananas).

It's important that kids are actually eating during their lunch break. We know it's easy for kids to end up studying during their lunch break making up a quiz, playing basketball, and a million things other than eating, but this pattern can lead to high hunger levels later on in the day that might be hard to manage. Check in with your teen on this. Are they actually having their lunch? Lunch carries them through their whole day. If they miss it, they will come home starving.

If you are packing their lunch, or preparing it in person, don't forget to include all food groups and make sure there is enough on the plate for your child to feel full.

"I was born in South Korea and came to the States when I was about five," said Dr. Norman Kim in a speech to the San Francisco Bay Area chapter of the International Association of Eating Disorders Professionals. "I have very clear memories of being horribly embarrassed that my lunch looked so different from all of the other kids' lunches, and that my mom didn't pack sandwiches because she didn't really know what a sandwich was. I would come to school with rice and a little bit of soup and food that smelled funny to other people. I remember how mortifying that experience was. I'd love it if anyone would pack me that kind of lunch today, but at the time it was very impactful. I think that is a very common experience that many of us (people of color) have."

Suggestions include:

- turkey sandwich with cheese and avocado, carrots, trail mix
- bean and cheese burrito, salad
- almond butter sandwich on whole-grain bread, with sliced banana inside, wheat thins on the side, yogurt
- pizza, salad with dressing
- grilled chicken salad (or tofu as the protein source), over greens, feta cheese, mixed vegetables, salad dressing, pita on the side
- ramen
- sushi rolls, edamame, salad.

What are some foods that are served in your household at this time of day?

_____

_____

_____

AFTERNOON SNACK

If you notice a pattern of your adolescent coming home from school feeling ravenous, a 1–2 on the Hunger Meter, it's important to assess what's happening so that you can break this pattern together. The goal is for them to come home less hungry. Eating to appetite is what we call a 3 on the Hunger Meter, the first sign of hunger. When your child arrives in a more peaceful place, ready to eat but not ravenous, they can eat more mindfully. They are also less likely to bypass their body's natural stopping place and figure out which foods they really want, rather than eating whatever they see in front of them. If your teen regularly comes home from school ravenous, you may want to explore the following with them:

- Did they skip a meal?

- Were their meals too small?

- Did they forget to bring a morning snack?

- Did their meals have all the food groups represented?

- Were their meals too boring or bland? Are they eating the same thing every day? (Sometimes boring meals will leave you looking for something exciting later on.)

- Was their energy expenditure different today? Did they have a harder workout? Do more in gym class today?

- Was something off from the day before? (It's possible this higher hunger could be from something that happened yesterday! A travel day, a higher workout load, or simply an "off eating day," might be catching up with them.)

Based on what you determine from the questions above, you will want to make changes, in order to help your teen get their hunger level up to a 3–4. For example, if they missed breakfast, brainstorm ways with your child to make sure breakfast can be included more regularly. Yes, this might involve setting the alarm for ten minutes earlier. A morning snack, in between breakfast and lunch, can offset a high hunger level and might be part of the plan; a bigger lunch might help, as well.

If the afternoon is the time when you expect to have hungry people walking in the door, it's good to be ready in advance. Discuss a plan with your kids, so you can have snacks waiting when they walk in the door. If your child is an athlete, the after-school snack will also serve as the pre-workout snack; this is important for fueling muscles during practice and giving them enough energy to compete. Some athletes go straight to practice after school, missing this important opportunity to fuel. Snacking after school, before practice, will not only help your child feel strong on the field but will also help them feel more in control of their hunger and fullness cues at dinner. Missing the afternoon snack could set your child up to overeat when they finally arrive home. Some delicious ideas at this time of day include:

Hunger Level 3

- apple or banana and peanut butter/almond butter/sunflower seed butter

- red pepper slices, whole grain crackers, and guacamole

- cookies and milk

- snap peas and guacamole

- granola bar and carrots

- brownie and milk

- yogurt, granola, strawberries

- smoothie (strawberries, banana, Greek yogurt, milk, ice)

- drinkable yogurt and pistachios

- blueberries and almonds

- trail mix and milk

- dark chocolate and cashews

- vegetable cutlets with chutney or other dipping sauce.

Hunger Level 4–5

- hummus, pita chips, and carrots

- avocado toast and egg

- smoothie (strawberries, banana, Greek yogurt, milk, ice) and protein powder

- falafel with dipping/tahini sauce

- half turkey sandwich or peanut butter and jelly sandwich (or whole depending on your appetite/energy needs)

- minestrone soup and crackers

- leftovers

- cheese and cracker plate with grapes.

What are some foods that are served in your household at this time of day?

_____

_____

_____

_____

_____

_____

DINNER

Dinnertime is a chance to relax after a long day, catch up with family, and eat together. Including a variety of different food groups will provide a filling and yummy meal for the whole family. Meal ideas include:

- chicken with rice, green beans, and a glass of milk

- taco night: ground turkey/beef/beans, salsa, cheese, lettuce, and tomato in a taco shell plus salad on the side

- burger night: beef/turkey/veggie patty, with bun, cheese, side salad

- salmon with green beans, brown rice, and a glass of milk

- rice bowl with black beans (or tofu, chicken, steak, fish), mixed peppers, salsa, avocado (or sour cream), cheese

- sesame tofu, brown rice, and broccoli, with a glass of soy milk

- spaghetti and meatballs (turkey, beef, or vegan) with parmesan cheese and tossed green salad with dressing

- butter chicken or paneer (homemade cheese) and veggie korma, rice, garlic naan or roti, yogurt

- daal, vegetable sabzi (vegetable dish), rice, naan or roti, yogurt

- pho

- beef and broccoli, rice, gyoza

- fried rice, oxtail soup, chopped yellow bell peppers and cucumbers, crispy kale (typical Indonesian dinner).

What are some foods that are served in your household at this time of day?

_____

_____

_____

_____

AFTER-DINNER SNACK/DESSERT

It's common to feel hungry a few hours after dinner. Many kids stay up late and may wish to add an after-dinner snack. Parents sometimes ask whether it is "bad" to eat at night. They may have heard they should stop eating at a certain time (oh, diet culture!). We like to think of this time as an "after-dinner snack." Sometimes, this snack will be dessert (dessert can also be served with dinner or at any other time of day,) and some of the time it might be something else. We want to empower parents to do what is aligned with their goals and values, given there is not a one-size-fits-all approach here. For example, one household may have a 6-year-old that has dinner and dessert at 6 p.m., then bedtime at 8. In the very same household, a 15-year-old sibling may have eaten the same dinner and dessert at 6 p.m., but is naturally off to bed later. In this case, the parent can support their teen in food-management strategies for an *equal in availability* snack break in the kitchen, away from school work.

For snack ideas, see the list of snacks above.

What desserts are common in your household?

_____

_____

_____

_____

_____

_____

Chapter 9

The Benefits of Boundaries

Your boundaries are not just about what you do or don't do. Your boundaries are really about forming. Boundaries form a person, they are around a person, they give you shape and definition.[1]

Randi Kreger, author of *Stop Walking on Eggshells*

Boundaries. We all need them. We *vaguely* know what they are. We remember reading that we should set some in our parenting, in order to raise healthy children. But what, exactly, are boundaries, why are they important, and how can we work in partnership with our teens to set and respect them? In this chapter, we are going to talk about techniques that you and your teen can use to improve boundaries and communication with each other (as well as the outside world!).

Developing good boundaries starts with you, the parent. But what if you grew up in a household where your boundaries were routinely broken, and you were taught to not make waves and to "just get along"? This can make it hard to know how to assert or define your own boundaries as a parent. Some of us were not always given a lot to work with, as kids ourselves, which makes it difficult to stand our own ground as adults and model appropriate boundaries for our children. When we speak the truth and bring our authentic selves to each conversation with our children, we can work on creating a healthy self, and therefore we will not be as likely to communicate through behaviors.

HOW DO WE START?

First and foremost, setting boundaries is about protecting your values, so in order to develop a boundary, a good starting place is knowing what you value.

Dr. Russ Harris, author of *The Happiness Trap*, states:

> Values are your heart's deepest desires for how you want to behave as a human being. Values are not about what you want to get or achieve; they are about how you want to behave or act on an ongoing basis. Keep in mind there are no such things as "right values" or "wrong values." It's a bit like our taste in pizza. If you prefer ham and pineapple, but I prefer salami and olives, that doesn't mean that my taste in pizza is *right* and yours is *wrong*. It just means we have different tastes. And similarly, we may have different values.[2]

EXPLORATION: Values List

What are the core values that define you as a person? Think of them as guiding principles. (For example, you might believe that it's always important to be truthful, no matter how hard it can be. Honesty, then, may be one of your deepest-held guiding principles.) We offer some prompts below, but we encourage you to use what fits best for you. You will also see some ideas about key areas in life. Add in areas that are right for you, and consider discussing your responses with a trusted person.

Compassion	Respect	Honesty	Efficiency	Kindness
Equity	Equality	Creativity	Dependability	Positivity

Loyalty	Transparency	Trust	Excellence	Authenticity
Humor	Optimism	Challenge	Integrity	Commitment

Family Relationships

▸ What type of spouse, child, sibling, family member, colleague, (insert relationship here) do you want to be?

▸ What are your guiding principles when it comes to the relationships in your life?

Example: (1) Patience. Because this is when we can really connect and get to know each other. (2) Honesty. Without real communication, we will never really understand one another.

Your example/practice example:

_____

Parenting

▸ What matters most to you when it comes to being a parent? What principles align with your ideal of parenting?

Example: Humor is a wonderful, often-overlooked guiding principle. Does humor play an important role in your parenting and overall family dynamic? Do you use humor to keep things relaxed during intense conversations?

Your example/practice example:

_____

_____

Body

▶ What are the core principles that shape (pun intended!) how you think about your body? Under ideal circumstances, how would you like to feel towards your body?

Example: (1) Respect. Without a foundation of respect, it's hard to build anything else, such as self-confidence. (2) Compassion, because when I'm too hard on myself compassion allows me to ease up and be my own friend.

Your example/practice example:

_____

_____

Food

▶ What type of relationship would you like to create with food? How would you like to behave in situations that are challenging in relation to food? If you could create a best-case scenario, what would that be?

Example: (1) Pleasure. Because enjoying food without stress adds joy to my life. (2) Contentment. Because meeting my needs (and wants) mindfully and intentionally allows me to be present and move on (in a good way).

Your example/practice example:

_____

_____

Other areas to consider: Work, Academics, Friendships, Wellness, Health, Rest and Relaxation, and so on.[3]

Your example/practice example:

_____

_____

If, in your household, you value all creatures' lives, you and your young children might have made a pact to rescue and rehab any injured backyard wildlife you've discovered across the years. However, you might all agree that while baby birds and squirrels are one thing, a hurt adult porcupine requires special attention and a phone call to Animal Services. Value, meet boundary.

If something is important to you, then it's important to teach other people about you. In other words, let them know your expectations. This gives them a choice. Someone else may value relaxation and have a different concept of time than you do. It doesn't mean they are wrong and you are right (remember those pizza toppings?), but it's important to not expect others to be just like us.

According to the Out of the FOG website, "Boundaries are about us getting clear inside of ourselves as to what is appropriate and necessary for our mental health, and then taking action accordingly."[4]

Sometimes people are going to exist or act in direct conflict with your values, wants, and needs, and that is okay because everyone is entitled to their own feelings, and that includes you. When someone is in direct conflict with you, it's important to not let it plant a seed of doubt. Hold tight to your confidence in your own values. Don't solely focus on keeping the peace outside of you; prioritize keeping the peace within yourself, as well.

The key is not to wait for a situation to take care of itself—it rarely does. We need to be proactive and speak up at the first sign of a problem, making boundaries click in a little bit earlier.

Most of us don't have a problem setting a boundary with a customer care provider when we've been charged for a product we didn't buy on our credit card, but somehow we have difficulty setting boundaries with people close to us. (Of course, this makes sense. It's much easier to assert ourselves with a stranger on the phone than with a friend, relative, or peer who is invading our personal boundaries.) Some may come from community or family traditions in which asserting oneself may be considered being too direct or even impolite. It can be challenging navigating situations like this. However, the principle on managing these situations is the same, asking yourself, "What are my core values?" In our experience, when people are out of alignment with their own values, they feel it, and it doesn't feel good. There may be times when you are not fully able to express what you want or do what you want as it relates to your core values in light of cultural or family expectations. That's okay. Awareness in these circumstances can become great learning moments and times for some self-reflection. By recognizing that something was off for you, you can think about if or how you want to do it differently should the situation come up again. Go back to the Value List exploration and think about what happened. What value did the incident touch for you?

Justyna on Boundaries Work

I didn't realize boundaries meant knowing myself more, and I thought I knew myself better. I don't think I ever really thought about what my boundaries are; I just know when certain things make me uncomfortable or that I don't like it. I will usually hold back, even if I want to say no or speak up for myself, out of fear of how the other person will respond. Emotional boundaries are a big one that I want to work on, because I still feel responsible for other people's feelings. When I am worried about hurting others, I stay in unhealthy situations too long or I'm taken advantage of.

Boundaries provide immense relief, offering us a better chance of positive and equitable relationships with our friends, family, and co-workers. For those of us who were raised to *not make waves*, at first setting boundaries can feel like robbing a bank. This does not mean the boundary is wrong; it just means you are breaking an old pattern (of people-pleasing). Don't give up—it gets easier over time.

When I first started really practicing boundaries, I felt HORRIBLE, because I got a lot of secondary gain out of people-pleasing, and knowing that I could find a way to get along with just about anyone. When I started speaking up for myself and setting boundaries in certain relationships, it was as if I lost that part of myself. Suddenly, people could be in direct conflict with me. Over time, I've honed the skill of "being okay with people not being okay with me." Remember: that horrible feeling in the beginning doesn't mean your boundary was wrong; it just takes time to lean into that discomfort. At first, I spent days worrying about my boundary—how it had been received, how the relationship might change, if I should have acted differently. Confidence in my own actions came with time. And, of course, some people are great at being held accountable and some... aren't. Don't let others' issues mess with you when you're a boundary-setting newbie; stick to your convictions (which are, after all, based on your values!).

—*Signe*

We can't count on people not pressing our buttons. During difficult times, like the pandemic (remember 2020), button-pushing felt like an inevitability. The key is to "dissolve your buttons." Really! Know your triggers. If you follow the trigger all the way down the rabbit hole and identify its source, what do you find? What can you learn from this trigger, and how can it help you establish a healthy boundary?

Let's walk this through. Say you are triggered by a family member who gives you unsolicited advice. Most of us are triggered by this; healthy emotional boundaries usually prevent us from giving unsolicited advice. And although most people might feel frustrated by this, the particular trigger is unique to each of us. One person might feel angry and disrespected, while another person may feel inadequate. Knowing what your trigger is (and bonus if you know where it comes from) will allow you to dissolve the trigger and undo its power.

Dr. Peter Levine, author of *Waking the Tiger: Healing Trauma*, states, "Traumatic symptoms are not caused by the 'triggering' event itself. They stem from the frozen residue of energy that has not been resolved and discharged."[5, 6] For example, let's say your uncle offered some unsolicited advice that left you feeling "white-hot," because you believe that inherent in his advice is the patronizing sense that he knows best. You feel disrespected. *How could he?* But here's the thing: your outrage may also be an indicator that you have some work to do when it comes to respectful relationships. The fact that you have unresolved respect issues means this is inevitably going to be a soft spot for you. Take this opportunity to bring that awareness into your own reaction to the unsolicited advice. Breathe. Express your boundary clearly and with confidence.

(While we're on the topic of advice: typically, if someone wants advice, they will ask for it. If they aren't asking, then you can safely assume they don't want it. If you do really want to dive in and offer ideas, it's good to request consent first—e.g. "Would it be okay to give feedback, or were you just needing to vent?")

CARING WITH DETACHMENT

Setting and maintaining boundaries with a teen is especially difficult, given that it's no fun to make our own child uncomfortable. We have a tendency to take on their pain, even though we can't actually regulate another person's emotions. And it doesn't serve anyone to carry your teen's problems around with you. The goal, instead, should be what Dr. Brenda Schaeffer, author of *Is It Love Or Is It Addiction?* calls "caring with detachment." This involves setting a healthy emotional boundary that lets you know where your teen ends and you begin.

Schaeffer states that we can care, listen, and respond to others' feelings, but we cannot "fix" or remove all ill feelings in others. Therefore, a sense of caring detachment is a healthy sign in a relationship. Parents say, "I care what you feel and I'm here for you," but not "Let me feel your pain for you," or "Let me help you feel better." Caring detachment is not indifference. You remain present to a person's pain, you are attentive, you let the person know you hear or support them, and you do not feel guilt or discomfort when you cannot do more.[7]

Empathy

Empathy is the ability to understand and share the feelings of another. Empathy is a strength, not a weakness; it is not something to "get rid of." Empathetic listening is basically being thoughtful or caring, as you listen to another. The challenge when expressing empathy is to maintain balance. It is important when listening to another person expressing their needs, that you don't lose sight of your own. Boundaries are key here, and in order to have boundaries, it would serve you to be clear on what your needs are and honor them.

—*Holly M. Davies, Intuitive Counselor*

Trust Me

Healthy relationships create a feeling of safety. This applies to the people in our lives as well as our relationship with ourselves. One of the characteristics that tell us someone is safe to trust is congruency. Congruency is making sure that our words and actions match. By being real with ourselves and others, we create transparency which builds trust. It's sort of like the "container" for our relationships. A pie pan is a metaphor for congruency; without the pan, the crust may hold for a little while, but eventually it will fall apart and all the ingredients for the pie will fall to the bottom of the oven. There can be no pie without the support of the pan!

PUTTING IT ALL TOGETHER

Developing healthy boundaries requires a willingness to name them for yourself, as well as the willingness to maintain them. While this skill may be difficult at the beginning (who among us hasn't forgone our own well-being in order to care for someone else?), without a solid understanding of our own limits, most of us end up feeling depleted and cranky.

Parenthood is defined by self-sacrifice and is often thankless. Particularly because of this, we encourage parents and caretakers to pause and allow themselves time and space to reflect on their own core values and guiding principles. Without clarity on what we actually want, we're likely expending a lot of energy doing things we don't want to, with people we don't really want to be with. Sound familiar?

Of course, there are absolutes. The kids have to be picked up from school. Cooking nutritious meals for your family is a priority for you. Fair enough! However, we encourage you to sit with the explorations in this chapter and revisit the Values List as you read your way through this book. When it comes to setting boundaries, there are no easy or quick fixes, but practice yields progress (if not perfection). And remember, your teen is watching. In setting your own compassionate boundaries, you're also modeling this valuable practice for your child.

EXPLORATION: Ad Libs for Effective Communication
(Goal: Mutual Respect)

Communicating effectively will vary depending on who you are communicating with. If you or your teen are in conflict with a peer, a good approach is to speak truthfully, because it matches your relationship. In this case, letting people know how you feel is an investment in the relationship. But what if the person you'd like to be assertive with is in a position of power? Perhaps it's your boss, or if you're a teen, maybe it's your parent? What if the person is unreasonable? The goal, then, would not be to speak truthfully, because you are afraid or don't know how, but rather to *choose* not to if that's what you decide. ("I have the skills to be forthcoming, but in this case, I'm choosing not to speak directly to... I know I cannot 'move' another person; I can only move myself.")

Sometimes, the less you say in response to verbal challenges, the better. The urge to defend can lead you directly into a circular conversation—arguments that go on almost endlessly, repeating the same patterns with no resolution. Short one-word responses can be most effective to keep yourself from being baited. You may also choose to state your position. Consider the exploration below as a skill set you can use to get prepared for a tough conversation, *or* use it to write out what you would have liked to have said but didn't feel comfortable saying. Just pouring out your thoughts in a journal—instead of keeping them bottled up inside—can be a very healthy response.

Example: Ad Libs for Effective Communication

"When you comment on my body without my consent, I feel angry, and hear in my mind that you are scrutinizing my body."

They say, "Well I just thought you looked great and wondered if you had lost weight."

You say, "That may be your perspective, but I wanted you to know how these comments affect me."

Exploration: Ad Libs for Effective Communication

"When you _____ (action), I feel _____ (feeling), and hear in my mind _____ (thought)."

They say _____

Follow up with your perspective _____

KNOWING YOUR INNER SELF

A key to having good boundaries is knowing your inner self: your values, wants, and needs. When you know your inner self, it's nearly impossible to be manipulated. If you are new to creating a healthy sense of self, have a variety of trustworthy friends and family write to you about what they think of you and what your strengths are. You'll find that most people will say the same things again and again. This can be a solution or a way to combat seeds of doubt. This can also be fun for parents to do for their teens. This practice will help your teen identify their values as well as the gifts they have to share. And heck, the adults could use this exercise every so often, too.

Chapter 10

Under the Influence of Social Media

Ninety-five percent of American teenagers now have access to a smartphone. Social media influencers are today's teen celebrities, with as much sway as movie stars. Information access is available at the touch of a button, with cutting-edge mobile phones having more capability than the first computers that launched humans into space. What does access to this much technology and information mean for character development, body image, personal boundaries, self-respect, and value formation?

That's a complex question, and the answer is not always clear. What is clear is that the responsibilities of parenting now include cyber security, stealthy information-accessing skills, and superhuman critical analysis of open-access global information that is created by everyone and their mother... literally. In short, parenting in the era of social media brings a whole new meaning to the word *complicated*.

Teens spend six to nine hours online in a typical day, and the pandemic further increased daily time spent on technology and devices. Sara Gilliam, co-author of *Reviving Ophelia: Saving the Selves of Adolescent Girls, 25th Anniversary Edition*, states, "We've let the train go shooting out of the station without pushing the brakes and thinking about how we can navigate the online world carefully and thoughtfully with our teenagers."[1]

In many ways, parents and guardians have already been run over by this train, because no one really taught anyone about this thing that became the world wide web, let alone how to navigate teenagers' (and our own!) obsession with social media. This is one of those bridges that we walked as it was built. And while technology has allowed us to explore, innovate, and gather online in ways we never have before, it has also enabled the creation of a second world, online, which can be problematic. In extreme cases, this virtual world can be harmful. A study examining media use over a ten-year period found that 13-year-old girls who used social media for 2–3 hours a day or more, and increased that use over time, had the highest levels of suicide risk in emerging adulthood.[2]

Gilliam recommends that parents sit down with their teenagers and really look at what their kids are doing online. She suggests: "You wouldn't let your kids spend that much time with a friend without having met the friend or their family."

Approach the online lives of your child with curiosity and ask them to give you a tour of their social media platforms. Ask specific questions such as, "Who are you following these days?" "What influencers do you like?" "What do you enjoy about them?"

Detailed questions may be annoying for your child, but they will also know that you're interested and that you're willing to ask. So ask. This is important not only for setting limits but also for your child's well-being and safety.

Parents should explore the apps and social media that their kids are using. This first-hand experience will help parents give advice and set ground rules around navigating the online world. If you're not familiar with the platforms, try out some of the things that your teen is doing. Make a video even if you don't post it. Ask your teen for help. Going through the motions may help you understand your teen's digital world. TikTok users have a "For You" page, which provides videos based on your teen's interests and past behaviors on the app. A general preview of content provides a valuable opportunity for you to experience and react to images, trends, sounds, social justice messages, inside jokes, and body image culture. Make sure your teen knows how and where they can report offensive or inappropriate content to moderators; this will allow them to use their voice. Once you have navigated this territory on your own, you will be positioned to engage in a deeper level of discussion with your teen.

When you take that deep dive, remind your teen that social media is filled with deceptive images that have been photoshopped, "Facetuned," filtered, or airbrushed. It is now common for adults and teens to spend considerable amounts of time trying to take the perfect selfie, and then filtering it to further refine the image. A report assessing media use, body dissatisfaction, and self-esteem found that many young women were obsessed with how many "likes" they were getting (and continued to check the number of post likes regularly), worried how they looked in their photos, and thought individuals would think they looked different on social media than in real life, all contributing to insecurities and increasing stress levels.[3] This slow slide from reality has caused many of us to miss out on what's actually happening right in front of us.

Without question, social media has upped the pressure on consumers to look a certain way and maintain a certain type of lifestyle, which may or may not match reality. Teens should be reminded that people post more of a "highlight reel" on their social media accounts, and almost never share about real life when they are having a bad day, are in a rotten mood, or are feeling uncomfortable in their skin. Social media breeds comparisons, and so inevitably teens will look on their feed and wonder why "everyone else is always happy," or "why everyone has so many friends," when they don't feel that same way. It's important to continue discussing together how social media does not reflect reality. Teens need a real understanding of what they are looking at, in order to adequately filter these comparisons and protect their self-esteem.

Teens also compare themselves to other images on social media, which can be further damaging to their self-esteem. A 2020 Common Sense Media survey found that the top two searches online by teens were for COVID-19 and fitness/exercise.[4] Teens may stumble on to "fitspo" and/or "thinspiration" influencers in minimal clothing showing off six-pack abs or chiseled biceps. These influencers appear to promote health and wellness, which might be appealing to image-conscious teenagers, but many of the messages celebrate diet culture. These messages often advocate for eating less, following fad diets, eliminating certain foods, or exercising in an unbalanced way. They put kids at high risk for the development of an eating disorder. We would recommend discussing these concerns with your teen, and ideally following trusted weight-inclusive, non-diet nutrition/health professionals instead.[5]

Our sense of how people look in real life can be warped by overexposure to these kinds of images. Research shows that images and lifestyles reflected in social media and online can increase one's feelings of inadequacy, and even brief exposure to provocative images can increase levels of body dissatisfaction, feelings of shame, and depression, lower self-esteem, and increase negative affect for all genders.[6,7,8,9] These effects can start young, too. A study published in March 2021 found that girls who played with "ultra-thin dolls" were more likely to want thin bodies than those who played with dolls with more diverse body types.[10] The authors concluded that body dissatisfaction can start in childhood and persist, becoming a risk factor for the development of eating disorders.

What is the best way to help your teen curate their social media feed, so they can feel connected to friends and generally positive about themselves? We tell our teens to stop following people who cause them to obsess more about their weight or body shape, or encourage them to change their appearance in any way. Invite your teens to undertake a social media detox and unfollow anyone who makes them feel bad. Instead, encourage your teen to follow people who inspire, motivate, and align more with their values. Have them follow influencers or individuals with diverse body shapes and sizes, from diverse racial and ethnic backgrounds, and from different parts of the world.

Additionally, help teens to expand their feeds to include other interests such as travel, pets, delicious cuisines, or craft ideas. Help them build perspective by showing them that a broader world exists beyond the culture of celebrity.

There can be benefits to social media, as well. These platforms can help teens connect with friends and family, raise awareness, and help facilitate comfortable and confiding spaces online to connect with others who are struggling with positive body image, eating disorders, identity, and sexuality. Teens, in particular, don't always feel safe confiding in their real-life communities, so the online sphere can be a helpful starting place. This is where online social communities can step in and serve as spaces where people can seek out support. For example, the National Eating Disorders Association prioritizes education as well as community connection through health affirming and pro-recovery content.[11]

Going on TikTok should be fun but when I go on TikTok for five hours, I feel lazy or unproductive. When I read a book, I feel good about myself even though both are passive forms of entertainment. TikTok is not necessarily an extremely bad way to spend time because I find it has helped me cultivate hobbies and learn new things. I've learned things about sewing, knitting, art, cooking, and even tips on cleaning that actually helped me clean my room recently. The issue is that, for me, TikTok is often used as a way to regulate my emotions. That is, when I feel stressed or anxious, I use it as a distraction or a break for my mind. I find it difficult to get off of the app and start doing something else even if I have something I need to do. This is probably due to the endless stream of content. For some reason, watching small one-minute videos in succession on TikTok is more interesting and stimulating for me than watching a TV show or movie I enjoy.

—*Lilah, 17-year-old*

Teens need structure with social media, just as they do with other aspects of their lives, such as academics, curfews, sleep, expectations of personal decency, and appropriate eating habits (relationship to food). Teens should be required to take breaks from electronic devices throughout each day. And don't panic: implementing small changes may not be difficult. In fact, many young people report being relieved when this practice of breaks is implemented. Building in non-tech time allows for time spent elsewhere, doing other things, and developing other interests away from social media.[12, 13]

Even if no "other" exploration happens, the experience of being bored can, in and of itself, be a useful and skill-building part of childhood. Constantly being a passive consumer of tech-driven images and sounds may dull the senses and facilitate apathy. It may also create a drive for getting back on a device as soon as possible. Being able to unplug and do nothing is not an act of laziness in the modern tech world; it is an acquired skill that has to be practiced. Can you sit and do nothing? No TV, no computer, no cell phone or tablet? Allow yourself time daily that is not task-oriented. Can you be with yourself without distraction and feel at ease? For how long? This is one of those instances in which parents modeling intentional, positive technology use will go a long way.

So turn off your tech and show your child what it means to unplug. If you find yourself struggling, ask yourself why turning off the tech is a challenge. The answers may not be simple and the exploration may feel uncomfortable, but we believe that you can do it! Remember that previous prompt about talking to your teen with curiosity? Do the same for yourself. This is a judgment-free zone. You're simply asking yourself about the competing priorities that keep you tethered to a device. And you're being self-reflective about whether you're using tech for coping, relaxing, checking out, or something else entirely. If these prompts and questions unmask some things you want to explore further, it may be worth a conversation with a trained professional or a trusted mentor.

Teens, adults, and even children now turn to their social media for advice on everything from dealing with break-ups to fixing their acne to finding healthy recipes and HIIT workouts. Let's all say it together: a Google search is not the same as medical expertise. Humans can be drawn to what's most sensational versus what's true or what's accurate. This tendency can be even more significant for teens. Teens may align with certain trends or fad diets to fit in socially. And while identifying with peers and being drawn to the latest trends are normal adolescent behaviors, in the context of social media they require extra intentionality.

In addition to personal awareness, we also recommend online information scrutiny. Teens should be invited to routinely question and be curious about content. Encourage them to think critically about the accuracy of the information they uncover. Learning to evaluate the credibility of an online source is a great step toward becoming a discerning consumer.

Let's be honest: there is some straight-up quackery on the internet. However, this same sensational content can be the most attractive. So if your teen's favorite celebrity or sports personality is saying something attention-grabbing, it's worth listening closely and looking twice.

The pull toward instant gratification and easy answers is compelling. Aligning with what validates our opinion can seem easiest, but can also be dangerous. For example, your teen might want a quick fix for an acne breakout. Looking online, they might find that a homemade honey and cinnamon mask will help. An expert might note that this may be soothing and could offer antibacterial effects, but there is very little evidence to support this claim. Yet a desperate teen could spend hours going down the rabbit hole of trying different online remedies without getting much benefit and, in some cases, possibly even aggravating the situation.

Snake-oil remedies existed long before the internet, but they weren't as easily available. There is great information available on adolescent-health-friendly websites (see resource section), but many sites may be propagating rumors and myths or peddling products. There's no way to get around that. Our goal isn't to stop all flow of online information or marketing. Rather, our aim is to help individuals, especially teens, become critical thinkers, so that they can make decisions that work for them based on current and accurate information.

In the case of acne, we like the Center for Young Women's Health (https://youngwomenshealth.org) and Young Men's Health (https://youngmenshealthsite.org). Even if you are looking for integrative medicine websites, outside of traditional medical models, reference national societies for credible links such as the Academy of Integrative Health and Medicine (https://aihm.org/vision) and the National Center for Complementary and Integrative Health (www.nccih.nih.gov).

Realistically, you are not going to be able to keep the young person in your home from encountering destructive messages from social media, their culture, or other kids, but you can help them to become critical consumers of media, as a way to build resilience within them and yourselves. Additionally, you can help them find great content online that will enhance their lives, rather than stymie them. One transformative way you and your teen can learn to become critical viewers of the media, right from the comfort of your own home, is through the movies you watch together.

Movies are also a fabulous way to discuss topics such as body image, defined by Marci Evans, R.D., as "an inner picture of your body and the way you feel about it."[14] The images we see on the screen affect the picture we have of our own body and the way we feel about it.

"Of course, not all films are created equal when it comes to looking critically at body image," Kristen Meinzer said. Meinzer is a culture critic and host of the podcast Movie Therapy with Rafer and Kristen:

> Even movies that shill themselves as size-inclusive have a tendency to make larger bodies the punchline (e.g. *Shallow Hal*, *The Nutty Professor*). Often, they put the protagonist on a weight-loss journey, where the happy ending is tied to the hero's new, smaller dress size (e.g. *Just Friends*, the TV show *Revenge Body*). Alternatively, they relegate the fat person to the role of funny, sassy, or wise best friend, whose only job is to help the thin protagonist self-actualize (e.g. *Pitch Perfect*, *Lady Bird*).

These messages are often subtle, but if we pay attention to the stories we are telling ourselves about these images, we can understand and challenge how they are influencing our lives and impressions. When our negative thoughts stay private, they can gain momentum. Films are a great way to encourage an appreciation for the diversity of bodies, and a whole lot more.

"Films that I think do a better job include *Last Holiday*, starring Queen Latifah; *Hairspray*, by John Waters; *Dumplin*, based on the book by Julie Murphy; the Pixar film *Up*; *Hidden Figures*, starring Octavia Spencer; and *Spy*, starring Melissa McCarthy. The list, while still lacking, is getting better every year," Meinzer said. "You just have to do your research. There are also a number of TV shows that depict diverse bodies in a fairly smart way: *Grey's Anatomy*, by Shonda Rhimes; *Shrill*, based on the book by Lindy West; *Sweet Magnolias*, based on the books by Sherryl Woods; and *Superstore* are just a few examples."

"In some of these films and TV shows, body acceptance is central to the plot," Meinzer added. "For example, in *Dumplin*, our fat protagonist of the same name enters a pageant as a 'protest in heels' to the superficial and narrow ideas of womanhood her mother and her community hold. In others, like *Grey's Anatomy* and *Superstore*, it's usually taken for granted that people come in a wide variety of sizes (as well as races and sexual orientations), just as in the real world. Still others, like *Spy* and *Last Holiday*, cast fat artists in the kind of Hollywood plots that traditionally center only thin people (action movie in the former case and romance in the latter); and then, transgressively, choose not to acknowledge the casting decision as unusual within the story, but instead treat it as a given."

Movie Therapy

Therapists have long recommended movies as a means of teaching mental health concepts and providing healing opportunities. This is called, somewhat irreverently, movie therapy. Movies can be comforting because they can show your teen that they are not the only ones suffering through the maturation process of adolescence (see any and all "coming of age stories," for example). Movies can open our eyes to important values, give glimpses into aspects of life we are exploring, such as setting boundaries or exploring first romantic relationships. Movies can be a cathartic way to release blocked emotions, too. (Have you ever seen a teenager try to hide their tears at the end of *Finding Nemo*?) Watching characters prevail over obstacles together can also help remind us that we are not alone.

Think about a personal growth topic you and your teen are currently exploring. Do you remember a movie that had a special impact on you during your teen years? Do you remember movies, characters, or film scenes that emotionally moved you? We encourage you to learn about a movie before watching it with the young people in your home. Reading the movie synopsis and checking out the Motion Picture Association of American (MPAA) or Common Sense Media rating is a good idea. Watch the movie ahead of time, so you can anticipate scenes that might be uncomfortable with your teen.

EXPLORATION

1. Pick a movie.

2. What about the movie matches what you are dealing with?

3. Who did you relate to in the movie and why?

4. Who did you have an aversion to and why?

5. Why is this movie significant to you? What does it mean to you?

THE TECH METER

Defining our personal values and ambitions is key to decision making—this was true long before the advent of the internet. Being a mindful consumer of technology is no different. Ingesting technology and media is similar to ingesting food: quality, quantity, and mindful use make a difference in well-being and personal outcomes. Regulated and intentional intake, mixed with mindful movement, thoughtful breaks, and other joyful activities, are just as relevant for tech use as they are for nutritional intake. Teens need a proactive approach to using technology and the "Tech Meter," similar to the "Hunger Meter," can help with personal awareness. This internal compass that is tuned to "tech-satiety" and "tech-hunger" is a vital personal tool (see graphic below). The goal is to allow for insight into "Where am I?" with my tech use (or overuse!).

A pause-and-reflect practice allows for space between habit and action. Individuals can make a conscious choice and engage with technology in a way that enriches their life. We encourage

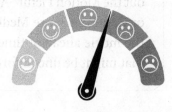

you to practice and apply the Tech Meter, in order to better understand yourself and your teen.

Level 1: Mindful and Limited Use

Individuals will likely use their technology at this level to complete focused tasks and perform essential functions. Maybe this is just log-in time to finish a school assignment or participate in meetings and remote education. At Level 1, you're using no more tech than is absolutely required. If you're content here, that's great...and atypical!

Level 2: Mindful and Content with Expanded Use

Level 2 is a good stopping place. You've completed work tasks. You've had a chance to connect with friends and family and spend some leisure time in your online world. You balance tech time with non-tech activities, such as reading or other hobbies. Tech is dialed down and turned off one or two hours before bed. Also, you engage in intentional offline activities and decisions for "no-use" time, such as during meals, family car trips, family outings, Saturday mornings, and so on. The point is that technology use is not disruptive to other aspects of your life and household.

Level 3: The Slippery Slope and Tiring Use

This is not a bad space to be in, especially if you've got a deadline or a report due and have to spend a little longer online. Likely, you've spent more time than you wanted to, and you might feel your eyes fatiguing and your mind tiring. If this is related to leisure time, you may be on yet another episode of an interesting show and know that it's time to stop, but talk yourself into "just one more." You're feeling anchored to the device and know that you don't like this feeling. You recognize that this isn't a good place to be, and consciously make an effort not to make this a regular practice. This zone is a slippery slope. Through repeated use and acclimation, this area can become the new normal if you're not frequently revisiting our central question: Where am I?

Level 4: Depleting Energy and Excessive Use

This is a bit of a gray area with progressive use. There may be a sense of preoccupation at this level, with an urge to repeatedly check your phone for email updates or social media updates. There may be a loss of time. You sat down to do something quickly and suddenly it's an hour later and you're watching rescue animal videos. It's not a loss of control, per se, but it's mindless engagement that spills over into excessive use. Perhaps you have a voice in your head asking, "Wait, why am I doing this?" This may be the point at which you start forgoing previously enjoyable activities in favor of time on screens or preferred technology. It may also be a point at which family members and friends point out that they want you to put down your phone or your tablet and give them your attention. Signs are pointing to the fact that you and those around you are a little concerned about how much technology you're using. We suspect that at this point, you are walking away after use more tired, not from the excess work but from the prolonged use.

Level 5: GIVE ME MY TECH!

At this level, we suspect that someone is highly driven to get to their go-to tech. This may be email or social media, gaming, a specific online channel, a streaming service, or something else. Usually, at this level you are craving tech. This can be due to a prolonged break from being on your preferred activity, feelings of boredom, or a desire to check out and relax. There can also be an obsessive quality that comes with this level.

There may be a seeking quality here as well. And as with any repetitive activity that we seek out during intense cravings, there may be negative consequences. While the activity may offer temporary relief, it may also lead to unintended impacts, such as missing deadlines, ignoring vital responsibilities, forgoing time with loved ones, and so on.

As with the Hunger Meter, we advocate for regulated tech intake through thoughtful planning, so that you do not overuse your various devices in a way that is harmful. We also recommend mindful reflection on how often you are hitting a point of seeking tech and craving tech to the point that it's interfering with life. Are you staying up until all hours to watch that next episode? Are you watching online videos about nothing yet are unable to log off? Are you playing your favorite game with no stopping point in sight, and to the extent that you are exhausted the next day?

EXPLORATION

Where are you on the Tech Meter?

Why?

DIGITAL AGREEMENTS

Align with your teen and their friends. Sara Gilliam suggests:

Invite teens to make *peer-to-peer agreements*. Be the family that hosts the pizza parties. Have your teen invite the kids they are on a group thread with to actually come hang out at the house. Encourage them to talk about agreements they can make that make their lives easier in regards to social media. Getting a group of kids to make agreements together as friends supporting each other is likely to have more staying power than rules from a parent or a school.[15]

We encourage you to talk to your teen about what is most relevant and pressing for them and their peer group. Are you hearing similar themes during the carpool or other times when your teen is talking to their friends? Do you hear problematic engagement such as online gossiping or mean texts about others?

Parents may also wish to discuss this important social media guideline with their teen: don't send or post images of yourself or other content that you wouldn't want to be splashed on the front page of a newspaper. We believe that people are empowered when they make choices. If teens want something to remain private, they should be vigilant about how they're sending it, and to whom. It's their content, but at the end of the day, they may no longer be in control of it. Are they okay with that? Is their family okay with that? Friends?

Example Peer-to-Peer Agreements

1. We don't look at our phones after 8 p.m.

2. You don't have to believe it! Support each other in questioning images and ideas of one way of being or thinking. If a friend sees a triggering image—for example, a body they perceive as better than theirs—we agree to have a dialogue, "Who says they have the right body and I have the wrong one? Where am I getting this message?"

3. Be inclusive. We agree not to target or exclude others. We agree not to hide behind screens and say hurtful things. We don't have to like everyone but we expect each other to be decent to one another.

4. What happens online stays online! We agree to be mindful about what content we post online and send to friends. This includes checking in with friends before posting photos of them.

EXPLORATION: Your Agreements

1. _____

_____

2. _____

_____

3. _____

_____

Chapter 11

Building a Friendship with Your Body

Friendship is the perfect metaphor for the relationship between body and food. A healthy friendship is generally defined by mutual respect, trust, joy, and good listening skills. Our best friendships bring out a true enjoyment of each other's company. The concept of friendship is abstract in some ways and concrete in others. If we extract these qualities and apply them to our relationship with food, it's easy to conclude that we don't have the healthiest friendship with food. Food is that friend who gets in your head and messes with your confidence, all while acting like your dearest ally (oh, and you can't live without this particular friend, even during your worst arguments!). This chapter takes aim at the unfriendly relationships many of us have with food and body. With support and knowledge, we can unpack and unburden ourselves of food-focused peccadillos we've grappled with across our own lifetimes, and over time establish long-lasting friendships with food. And just in time, because our teenagers need all the support they can get as they grow into confident, capable young adults, rooted in healthy body image.

BODY IMAGE ON A SPECTRUM

The way we feel about our bodies spans along a continuum and often changes from day to day. Eating disorders specialist and sport psychologist Riley Nickols, Ph.D., notes:

> Body image is often framed as a black-and-white issue: either you feel good about your body, or you don't. The reality, however, looks more like a spectrum. On the negative and unwholesome end of the spectrum, your body image can be critical, evaluative, and distressing. You may fixate on perceived flaws, and spend a disproportionate amount of time thinking about the ways you need to change your diet, exercise routine, or other habits to fix them. "Disproportionate" can't necessarily be defined as a number or percentage of minutes or hours, but rather the degree of interference it has on your thoughts, actions, and behaviors. On the positive and wholesome end of the body image spectrum, someone might feel confident and accepting with their body's shape and size, secure and comfortable in their skin, and recognize that physical appearance is just one part of their identity.

These feelings can change based on our mood, events of the day, and environment. We have seen body image worsen for teens during finals week and improve during vacation. Likewise, your teen might feel one way about their body in the locker room and a different way entirely when out with their friends on a Friday night.

STRATEGIES FOR IMPROVING BODY IMAGE

We will discuss a few ways that you and your teen can work on improving their friendship with their body. These skills take practice but, over time, they will help them find more peace.

Treat Your Body with Respect

We are bound to fall out of "like" with our friends at times, given we aren't clones of each other. But if we can treat them with respect, even when we don't like them, we will find a quicker return to our baseline relationship with them. Apply the same principle to body image. Sometimes it's hard to even tolerate our body; self-judgment is high and self-tolerance is low. The willingness to practice kindness is a staple of a mutually respectful relationship. Your good friends will always have your back, and your body does, too. It's especially important to treat ourselves with compassion during tough times. Treating ourselves well, even in difficult moments, is a key skill for establishing a friendship with food and body.

Expand Your Definition of Beauty

Within every culture, there tends to exist a beauty ideal. The Body Positive (TBP) helps people develop balanced, joyful self-care and a relationship with their bodies that is guided by love, forgiveness, and humor. They encourage us to recognize that beauty is not the problem; the problem is the narrow definition of beauty and the exclusion that these limited ideas create. TBP co-founder Elizabeth Scott states, "The goal is to expand our definition of beauty to include ourselves and our ancestors as they show up in our bodies." People of all shapes and sizes can have a positive body image and a healthy respect for themselves. However, many cultures force the idea that those who don't look a certain way shouldn't feel positive about who they are. By rejecting constricted ideas of beauty and expanding the definition of what it means to be someone who is thriving and appreciative of their physical appearance, we not only decrease our personal stress but also create a more inclusive paradigm.

Reduce "Body-checking" Behaviors

Body checking refers to pinching different parts of one's body, pulling, squeezing, obsessing about your reflection in the mirror, looking at old photos, trying on old clothes that used to fit, or comparing yourself with other people. During the rise of virtual meetings and online school, we also saw an increased incidence of "zoom checking" or "face checking," in which people were focused on the way their face or individual features—their eyes, chin, and so on—looked. Body checking may also include asking others about their weight, shape, or appearance, in an effort to gain feedback or even validation. There is never an answer that will be satisfying: scrutiny breeds dissatisfaction. If we are looking for flaws, we're going to find them. Those who body check, even after positive feedback, rarely walk away feeling good. Body checking is shown to increase feelings of depression and anxiety, and feelings of loss of control around shape and weight.[1]

The first step to reducing body checking is to tune in to these behaviors. (How many times during that video call did I reposition my camera to improve the angle? Why do I keep making myself try on the same pair of pre-childbirth jeans? What am I gaining from that experience?) Since we know that body-checking behaviors are net negative, it's then time to spring into action and implement strategies that will help us reduce body-checking behaviors in our daily lives. You can interrupt a bad body image thought simply by using a "stop technique" which sounds like: "This behavior/thought is not in my best interest, I'll stop obsessing this instant." That way, it literally "cuts the cord" to the thought. If someone is still body checking, rather than saying something negative when they look in the mirror, "redefine the narrative" with something more empowering. For example, a dancer was struggling with her body image, and reminded herself that "these are the legs that help me to leap through the air."

Some of us might need to get rid of mirrors for a while if we can't quit compulsively evaluating our appearance. Others should stop comparing their current selves with old photos and may need to delete or pack away said photos. Closing the Zoom video may provide relief for those of us who are unable to be kind and loving to ourselves during the workday. Finally, sharing your goal of reducing these behaviors with a loved one can help! Invite them to gently "interfere" when they notice you body checking unconsciously.

Body checking looks different for everyone. Here is one teen's description of her body image concerns:

Every reflective surface I see, I look at myself, suck in my stomach, and study my image. Someone might think I am vain, but really it's the opposite; I am terribly insecure about how I look and obsessed with every detail about my appearance. My friends are white, blonde, blue-eyed, and stick thin. I am more curvy, hour-glass shaped, and brown-skinned. The constant comparison I impose on myself makes me think something is wrong with me.

EXPLORATION: 24-hour Body-checking Surveillance

Clients will often say to us, "I don't think I engage in body-checking behaviors." But once they become aware of what body checking is, they often realize they are engaging in these kinds of behaviors without even knowing it. One definition of *habit* is "something a person starts doing before realizing they are doing it."[2]

The goal of this exploration is to increase awareness of

body-checking behaviors by tracking them over a 24-hour period (and no, you do not need to track while you sleep, although bonus points if you figure out how to do so!). Use the chart below to gain insight on when and if you or your teen are body checking, how frequently this may be occurring, and how this makes you or your teen feel (be prepared: it's not typically a mood enhancer!). Awareness gives you a choice; consider the formula "Awareness + Action = Change."

Example Exploration

24-hour Body-checking Surveillance		
Time of Day	Behavior	Feelings
6:30 a.m.	Tried on old jeans while getting ready for work	Depressed, they don't fit
7:00 a.m.	Pinched stomach area	Stressed
7:05 a.m.	Looked at a photo of me wearing those jeans	Disappointed

Practice Exploration

24-hour Body-checking Surveillance		
Time of Day	Behavior	Feelings

Diversify Interests

Peer identification and the desire to fit into a social group is a key part of adolescent development. It's normal for teens to experiment with their clothes, hair, make-up, or speaking style, among other things, as they explore the question, "Who am I?" Balancing being different and fitting in is a high-stakes game during adolescence. So, even though most teens are testing boundaries and trying to express their unique senses of self, they're usually doing it through the filter of the latest, peer-approved trends. In other words, teens who want to be unique will often try to dress or speak like their friends.

The very typical adolescent trait of over-identification with peers can lead to an intense dependence on a social group. This intensity is normal and can be particularly common among enthusiastic athletes, for example. The teen athlete may live, breathe, and dream about their sport—at the expense of school, family, other friendships, and almost everything else. But if the teen is cut from the team or injured, their world may quickly crumble. It's like having a house full of plants but only watering one of them, *all the time*. You will kill that one as well as the others.

Sport psychologist Riley Nickols explains:

> Deriving value from your sport participation can be healthy, but if you over-identify with your athlete identity, you're making a good thing an "ultimate" thing. In other words, if all of your worth comes disproportionately from a singular domain in your life, whether it's your role in school as a learner or your athleticism, any threat to those domains has the potential to destabilize you.

Nickols goes on to say:

> Ideally you want to hold these identities in your "mind's eye" more abstractly so that you can have security that this identity

is preserved and not entirely dependent on circumstances. For example, "I know that I am a son even though my parents aren't currently with me at the present moment." For the teen, an example of a resilient, non-contingent identity might be "I'm intelligent, even though I did poorly on that last test" or "Having a stress fracture and needing to take a break in my sport doesn't make me any less of an athlete." Specific to body image dissatisfaction, not only is it an unhealthy domain, it can also impair sport performance and be interfering across all domains of life. Expanding one's identity to be more inclusive and representative of the uniquely nuanced personality traits, dispositions, and skill sets that we possess as humans is both protective and preventative against developing a unidimensional identity.

Keep It Micro

If you are convinced that you'll never love your body no matter what you do, you won't be motivated to change your own mind. Conversely, having hope that something can change is enough to make change happen over time.

"Hope is the only positive emotion that needs negativity or uncertainty," wrote Dan Tomasulo in his book *Learned Hopefulness*.[3] He explains that even the tiniest feeling of wanting something new, or being able to envision it, is enough to initiate a change. "It's like a match, or when you light something, it starts a little bit and then it takes off."[4]

Smaller goals keep us motivated, engaged, and connected to the larger goals we're after. Rather than "love your body," which might feel daunting as a starting place if there's a fair amount of body hate, Tomasulo suggests micro-goals to improve body image. The more calibrated the goal, the better the outcome. If you feel an inkling of hope that change can happen, then you feel a sense of achievement from it—for example, "I've changed my perception of my body image for 60 seconds." Believe it or not, a micro-goal can be empowering and infectious. Other examples of micro-goals Tomasulo also mentions include a pause in negative thinking about your body, for example, a simple in-breath saying: "I accept this is my body," followed by an out-breath, "and I'm ready for change," would give a slight, intentional pause, to the negativity.[5] He states that by repeating this small goal, you can extend a single cycle of this in- and out-breath to a minute. A micro-goal can naturally lead to the next challenge.

One client Signe worked with aimed to simply "not hate" her body for three minutes each day. It was a surprisingly effective initial micro-goal that laid the groundwork for long-term progress toward her larger goals of self-acceptance and peace.

Using a Hopeful Mindset

- I will always hate my body, there is no way I will ever be okay with it, and I cannot see that ever changing.

- It's hard to imagine ever being okay with my body, but I'm open to trying. What is my next step?

Notice the difference between these statements? One is an example of a mindset without hope, and the other is an example of a hopeful mindset. Actualizing a hopeful mindset, even for a short period of time, can and will help you or your teen make positive progress over time. For example, try this:

I will commit to 60 seconds daily of intentional thought about times when I've had an appreciation for what my body has done for me. I can recall a period of time when I was training to hike Half Dome. I felt strong during that time, which boosted my body image, despite the fact it did not change my body/size. I notice that now that I've been able to change my perception for 60 seconds, maybe I've been wrong?

PRACTICE: MINDSET WITHOUT HOPE VERSUS HOPEFUL MINDSET

Mindset without hope:

_____

_____

_____

Hopeful mindset:

_____

_____

_____

COMMON BODY IMAGE QUESTIONS AND ANSWERS

We spoke to Virginia Sole-Smith, author of the book _The Eating Instinct: Food Culture, Body Image, and Guilt in America_ and the newsletter Burnt Toast, about common questions we hear from parents. She pretty much rocked the interview.

What do I say when my teen says they feel fat?

Sole-Smith: First, validate their experience of struggling in their body: "I'm so sorry you aren't feeling good about yourself right now. That is really hard." Then ask them to tell you more about their frustrations. Your goal is to gently guide them to understanding that "fat" is not a feeling; it's a word we use to mask underlying feelings. So maybe they're feeling anxious about an upcoming event and channeling that anxiety on to their body. Maybe they're feeling depressed. Encourage them to dig deeper and explore those emotions, and offer whatever support you can to help them navigate that. But be sure to emphasize that they do not need to change their body—and also that changing their body will not resolve the underlying feelings.

What do I say when my teen asks me, "Am I fat?"

Sole-Smith: If your teen asks if they're fat, and you can tell that maybe they think fat is a bad thing, the most important thing you can do is let them know that you accept their body—no matter what its size. You can say, "There's nothing wrong with being fat. Your body is never the problem. I never want you to make yourself smaller. I want you to take up all the space you need in the world."

What do I say when my teen talks about their friends who are dieting?

Sole-Smith: If your teen comes home from school talking about a friend on a diet, you might say something like, "Her body is not the problem. I'm sad her doctor told her to diet because I don't think anybody needs to make themselves smaller."

How do I explain fatphobia to my teen?

Sole-Smith: You can start by casually pointing it out whenever you see it. Pop culture is always so helpful that way! "I'd forgotten that these old episodes of *Friends* have so much fatphobia. I hate how they shame Monica for being fat in high school. There's nothing wrong with being fat." You can also start to talk about how fatphobia manifests in the systemic oppression of people in larger bodies. Research shows that fat people receive inadequate medical care and are discriminated against in schools and on job interviews. Even pointing out ways the physical world isn't built for fat bodies—seats in restaurants, airplanes, clothing stores—can be useful.

Conclusion

The teen years are about change. In reality, that's true for life across the spectrum. However, the adolescent years can be more expansive, defined by the desire to explore and experience life. These wonder years are usually filled with awkwardness, change, and a desire for independence that is an interesting combination of hope and positivity. They are also a pivotal time during which young people are individuating, building their identity, and establishing core values and guiding principles. Foundational pieces such as a rich sense of self and a solid friendship with food and body are at the heart of lifelong health and happiness. Parenthood and "guardianhood" are not easy. Caretakers are challenged on a day-to-day and sometimes moment-to-moment basis to respond to new and sometimes befuddling situations. Of course, all of this is happening as they (we) are navigating our own health and well-being and multiple competing priorities.

In our book *No Weigh! A Teen's Guide to Positive Body Image, Food, and Emotional Wisdom*,[1] we wrote:

Our goal continues to be to provide you with tools that give you more knowledge and a broader view of nutrition and well-being. Always go back to the basics, make time for yourself. Eat and enjoy everything with a strong foundation of balance. Make choices that work for you and that have also been shown to be scientifically critical, such as having a regulated sleep schedule, turning off the tech, and letting your mind power down. Be mindful and willing to take a moment to really feel your feelings, hone in on hunger cues or emotional cues, and identify what the true need is in that moment. Step into the solution...

That really sums it up.

We hope that this book has helped you to better understand your teen. We also hope that it has supported you in gaining personal insight through knowledge and reflective exercises. We encourage you to have a daily practice of well-being so that you can truly give to others that which you have for yourself—health and wellness. We encourage you to reference and return to this book and the explorations as often as you need to. We wish you an enduring friendship with food and body.

Resources

SUNNY SIDE UP NUTRITION WEBSITE AND PODCAST

Sunny Side Up Nutrition is a resource for parents about family feeding, nutrition, and simple cooking, free of diet culture. Sunny Side Up Nutrition (**www.sunnysideupnutrition.com**) offers parents advice on how to approach food in their home, resources, and very easy recipes. Sunny Side Up Nutrition also has a podcast with topics about raising children to eat well and feel good about their bodies! The podcast can be found on your podcast app!

THE BODY POSITIVE

Since 1996, The Body Positive (**www.thebodypositive.org**) has been offering experiential, online leadership training for initiating powerful Be Body Positive programs in middle schools, high schools, colleges, and community programs. Their compelling training and research-supported curriculum prepare both youth leaders and adults to establish an environment (either in person or online) for students to bravely explore their beauty, health, and identity, and the societal conditions that can lead to disruptions in embodiment. The Be Body Positive Model helps all people develop balanced, joyful self-care and a relationship with their bodies that is guided by love, forgiveness, and humor. Contact: info@thebodypositive.org or **https://thebodypositive.org**.

NATIONAL EATING DISORDERS ASSOCIATION (NEDA)

NEDA supports individuals and families affected by eating disorders and serves as a catalyst for prevention, cures, and access to quality care. Are you worried that you or someone you care about is struggling with an eating disorder? Early detection and intervention are key to recovery. Use NEDA's free and confidential screening to learn if it is time to seek professional help: **www.nationaleatingdisorders.org/screening-tool**.

For treatment options, visit **www.nationaleatingdisorders.org** or contact NEDA's Helpline: 1-800-931-2237.

THERAPY ROCKS! A PERSONAL GROWTH PODCAST

Therapy Rocks! The road to self-discovery is long, winding, and often complicated to navigate alone. Fasten your seat belt and join psychotherapist Signe Darpinian in conversation with a diverse roster of guests as they fearlessly explore all things human. With topics ranging from body image to sleep to the quest for the answers to our constant digital connectedness and more. This monthly podcast seeks out and celebrates both the humor and pathos encountered as we strive for personal growth in a wildly imperfect world. **www.signedarpinian.com/podcast**

Endnotes

Chapter 1

1   Loud, K.J. and Gordon, C.M. (2006) Adolescent bone health. *Archives of Pediatric and Adolescent Medicine 160*, 10, 1026-1032. doi:10.1001/archpedi.160.10.1026.

2   Kueper, J., Beyth, S., Liebergal, M., Kaplan, L., and Schroeder, J.E. (2015) Evidence for the adverse effect of starvation on bone quality: A review of the literature. *International Journal of Endocrinology.* doi:10.1155/2015/628740.

Chapter 2

1   Nakao, M. (2019) Heart rate variability and perceived stress as measurements of relaxation response. *Journal of Clinical Medicine 8*, 10, 1704. doi:10.3390/jcm8101704.

2   Arch, J.J. and Craske, M.G. (2006) Mechanisms of mindfulness: Emotion regulation following a focused breathing induction. *Behaviour Research and Therapy 44*, 1849-1858. doi:10.1016/j.brat.2005.12.007.

3   Seppälä, E.M., Nitschke, J.B., Tudorascu, D.L., Hayes, A., *et al.* (2014) Breathing-based meditation decreases posttraumatic stress disorder symptoms in U.S. military veterans: A randomized controlled longitudinal study. *Journal of Traumatic Stress 27*, 4, 397-405. doi:10.1002/jts.21936.

Chapter 3

1   Maas, J.B. and Robbins, R.S. (2011) *Sleep for Success: Everything You Must Know About Sleep But Are Too Tired to Ask.* Bloomington, IN: AuthorHouse.

2   Suni, E. (2020) Nutrition and Sleep. Accessed on 8/9/2021 at www.sleepfoundation.org/nutrition.

3   Roehrs, T.A., Burduvall, E., Bonahoom, A., Drake, C., and Roth, T. (2004) Ethanol and sleep loss: A "dose" comparison of impairing effects. *Sleep 26*, 8, 981-985. doi:10.1093/sleep/26.8.981.

4   Suni, E. (2020) Teens and Sleep. Accessed on 8/9/2021 at www.sleepfoundation.org/teens-and-sleep.

5   Centers for Disease Control and Prevention (2020) WISQARS™—Web-based Injury Statistics Query and Reporting System. Accessed on 8/9/2021 at www.cdc.gov/injury/wisqars/index.html.

6   Walker, M. and McGonigal, K. (2020, December 8) Underslept and Idle: The Transformative Effects of Sleep and Movement, Matthew Walker, PhD, in conversation with Kelly McGonigal, PhD. Accessed on 8/9/2021 at www.commongroundspeakerseries.org/matthew-walker-and-kelly-mcgonigal.

7   Shapiro, C.M. (1981) Sleep and the athlete. *British Journal of Sports Medicine 15*, 1, 51–55. doi:10.1136/bjsm.15.1.51.

8   Cohen, D.A., Wang, W., Wyatt, J.K., Kronauer, R.E., *et al.* (2010) Uncovering residual effects of chronic sleep loss on human performance. *Science Translational Medicine 2*, 14, 14ra3. doi:10.1126/scitranslmed.3000458.

9   American Academy of Sleep Medicine. (2008, June 10). Extra Sleep Improves Athletic Performance. Accessed on 8/9/2021 at www.sciencedaily.com/releases/2008/06/080609071106.

10 Cowley, L. (2017) The impact of sleep on athletic performance. Accessed on 8/9/2021 at https://elitetrack.com/impact-sleep-athletic-performance-lauren-cowley.

11 Mah, C.D., Mah, K.E., Kezirian, E.J., and Dement, W.C. (2011) The effects of sleep extension on the athletic performance of collegiate basketball players. *Sleep 34*, 7, 943–950. doi:10.5665/sleep.1132.

12 Milewski, M.D., Skaggs, D.L., Bishop, G.A., Pace, J.L., *et al.* (2014) Chronic lack of sleep is associated with increased sports injuries in adolescent athletes. *Journal of Pediatric Orthopaedics 34*, 2, 129–133. doi:10.1097/BPO.0000000000000151.

13 Lebron James: Daily Routine. Accessed on 8/9/2021 at www.balancethegrind.com.au/daily-routines/lebron-james-daily-routine.

14 Darpinian, S. (2021, March 28) How Optimizing Sleep Optimizes Well-Being. Therapy Rocks! Episode 14. Accessed on 8/9/2021 at https://audioboom.com/posts/7832530-how-optimizing-sleep-optimizes-well-being.

15 Prather, A.A., Janicki-Deverts, D., Hall, M.H., and Cohen S. (2015) Behaviorally assessed sleep and susceptibility to the common cold. *Sleep 38*, 9, 1353–1359. doi:10.5665/sleep.4968.

16 Walker, M. (2017) *Why We Sleep: Unlocking the Power of Sleep and Dreams.* New York, NY: Scribner (pp.311–312).

17 University of Granada (2011, November 22) Adolescents who sleep better score higher in math and physical education. ScienceDaily. Accessed on 8/9/2021 at swww.sciencedaily.com/releases/2011/10/111020025758.htm.

18 Gruber, R., Somerville, G., Enros, P., Paquin, S., Kestler, M., and Gillies-Poitras, E. (2014) Sleep efficiency (but not sleep duration) of healthy school-age children is associated with grades in math and languages. *Sleep Medicine 15*, 12, 1517–1525. doi:10.1016/j.sleep.2014.08.009.

19 Axelsson, J., Sundelin, T., Ingre, M., Van Someren, E.J., Olsson, A., and Lekander M. (2010) Beauty sleep: Experimental study on the perceived

health and attractiveness of sleep deprived people. *BMJ 341*, c6614. doi:10.1136/bmj.c6614.

20 Oyetakin-White, P., Suggs, A., Koo, B., Matsui, M.S., *et al.* (2015) Does poor sleep quality affect skin ageing? *Clinical and Experimental Dermatology 40*, 1, 17–22. doi:10.1111/ced.12455.

21 Schrom, K.P., Ahsanuddin, S., Baechtold, M., Tripathi, R., Ramser, A., and Baron, E. (2019) Acne severity and sleep quality in adults. *Clocks and Sleep 1*, 4, 510–516. doi:10.3390/clockssleep1040039.

22 Baiden, P., Tadeo, S.K., and Peters, K.E. (2019) The association between excessive screen-time behaviors and insufficient sleep among adolescents: Findings from the 2017 youth risk behavior surveillance system. *Psychiatry Research 281*, 112586. doi:10.1016/j.psychres.2019.112586.

23 Common Sense (2015) *The Common Sense Census: Media Use by Tweens and Teens*. San Francisco, CA: Common Sense Media. Accessed on 8/9/2021 at www.commonsensemedia.org/sites/default/files/uploads/research/census_executivesummary.pdf.

24 Alutaybi, A., Al-Thani, D., McAlaney, J., and Ali, R. (2020) Combating Fear of Missing Out (FoMO) on social media: The FoMO-R Method. *International Journal of Environmental Research and Public Health 17*, 17, 6128. doi:10.3390/ijerph17176128.

25 Ostrin, L.A., Abbott, K.S., and Queener, H.M. (2017) Attenuation of short wavelengths alters sleep and the ipRGC pupil response. *Ophthalmic and Physiological Optics 37*, 4, 440–450. doi:10.1111/opo.12385.

26 360 Research Reports (2019) Global blue light blocking glasses market 2019 by manufacturers, regions, type and application, forecast to 2024. Accessed on 8/23/2021 at www.360researchreports.com/global-blue-light-blocking-glasses-market-14357890.

27 Foley, L. (2021) Caffeine and Sleep. Accessed on 8/9/2021 at www.sleepfoundation.org/nutrition/caffeine-and-sleep.

28 World Health Organization (n.d.) Drugs (psychoactive). Accessed on 8/9/2021 at www.who.int/health-topics/drugs-psychoactive#tab=tab_1.

29 Ribeiro, J.A. and Sebastião, A.M. (2010) Caffeine and adenosine. *Journal of Alzheimer's Disease 20*, s1, S3–s15. doi:10.3233/JAD-2010-1379.

30 Chaudhary, N.S., Grandner, M.A., Jackson, N.J., and Chakravorty, S. (2016) Caffeine consumption, insomnia, and sleep duration: Results from a nationally representative sample. *Nutrition 32*, 11–12, 1193–1199. doi:10.1016/j.nut.2016.04.005.

31 Tanner, L. (2014, February 10) Caffeine consumption, mainly from soda, common in kids and teens. Associated Press. Accessed on 2/12/2018 at www.nydailynews. com/life-style/health/kids-teens-regular-caffeine-buzz-study-article-1.1608612.

32 Center for Behavioral Health Statistics and Quality (2020) *2019 National Survey on Drug Use and Health: Detailed Tables*. Rockville, MD: Substance Abuse and Mental Health Services Administration.

33 Centers for Disease Control and Prevention (2020) Youth Risk Behavior Surveillance—United States, 2019. *Morbidity and Mortality Weekly Report*, Supplement, 69, 1, 1–83.

34 Centers for Disease Control and Prevention (2020) Underage Drinking. Accessed on 8/9/2021 at www.cdc.gov/alcohol/fact-sheets/underage-drinking.htm.

35 Maas, J.B. and Robbins, R.S. (2011) *Sleep for Success: Everything You Must Know About Sleep But Are Too Tired to Ask*. Bloomington, IN: AuthorHouse.

36 Walker, M. (2017) *Why We Sleep: Unlocking the Power of Sleep and Dreams*. New York, NY: Scribner

37 Walker, M. (2021, May 27) The buzz on alcohol and caffeine. MasterClass. Accessed on 8/23/2021 at www.masterclass.com/classes/matthew-walker-teaches-the-science-of-better-sleep/chapters/the-buzz-on-alcohol-and-caffeine.

38 Nicholson, A.N., Turner, C., Stone, B.M., and Robson, P.J. (2004) Effect of Delta-9-tetrahydrocannabinol and cannabidiol on nocturnal sleep and early-morning behavior in young adults. *Journal of Clinical Psychopharmacology 24*, 3, 305–313. doi:10.1097/01.jcp.0000125688.05091.8f.

39 Winiger, E.A., Huggett, S.B., Hatoum, A.S., Friedman, N.P., *et al.* (2020) Onset of regular cannabis use and young adult insomnia: An analysis of shared genetic liability. *Sleep 43*, 5, zsz293. doi:10.1093/sleep/zsz293.

40 National Institute on Drug Abuse (2021) What are marijuana's long-term effects on the brain? Accessed on 8/9/2021 at www.drugabuse.gov/publications/research-reports/marijuana/what-are-marijuanas-long-term-effects-brain.

41 Shen, H. (2020) News Feature: Cannabis and the adolescent brain. *Proceedings of the National Academy of Sciences 117*, 1, 7–11. doi:10.1073/pnas.1920325116.

42 Jacobus, J. and Tapert, S.F. (2014) Effects of cannabis on the adolescent brain. *Current Pharmaceutical Design 20*, 13, 2186–2193. doi:10.2174/13816128113199990426.

43 Mozes, A. (2017) How much melatonin is really in that supplement? WebMD. Accessed on 8/9/2021 at www.webmd.com/sleep-disorders/news/20170301/how-much-melatonin-is-really-in-that-supplement.

44 Erland, L.A. and Saxena, P.K. (2017) Melatonin natural health products and supplements: Presence of serotonin and significant variability of melatonin content. *Journal of Clinical Sleep Medicine 13*, 2, 275–281. doi:10.5664/jcsm.6462.

45 Walker, M. (n.d.) Matthew Walker Teaches the Science of Better Sleep. Accessed on 9/8/2021 at www.masterclass.com/classes/matthew-walker-teaches-the-science-of-better-sleep.

46 Insomnia Severity Index (n.d.) Accessed on 9/8/2021 at www.ons.org/sites/default/files/InsomniaSeverityIndex_ISI.pdf.

47 Headspace (2021) How to build a perfect wind-down routine. Accessed on 8/9/2021 at www.headspace.com/blog/2019/03/27/sleep-health-3-how-to-build-a-perfect-wind-down-routine.

Chapter 4

1 Barry, V.W., Baruth, M., Beets, M.W., Durstine, J.L., Liu, J., and Blair, S.N. (2014) Fitness vs. fatness on all-cause mortality: A meta-analysis. *Progress in Cardiovascular Diseases 56*, 4, 382–390.

2 Women's Sports Foundation (n.d.) Our Research. Accessed on 8/9/2021 at www.womenssportsfoundation.org/what-we-do/wsf-research.

3 Women's Running (n.d.) This is How You Raise Healthy Female Athletes. Accessed on 8/9/2021 at www.womensrunning.com/health/wellness/raising-healthy-female-athletes.

4 *The New York Times* (2019) Why so many of us don't lose weight when we exercise. Accessed on 8/9/2021 at www.nytimes.com/2019/07/03/well/move/weight-loss-gain-exercise.html

5 Mountjoy, M., Sundgot-Borgen, J., Burke, L., Carter, S., *et al.* (2014) The IOC consensus statement: Beyond the Female Athlete Triad—Relative Energy Deficiency in Sports (RED-S). *British Journal of Sports Medicine 48*, 7, 491–497. doi:10.1136/bjsports-2014-093502.

6 Sobczak, C. (2014) *Embody: Learning to Love Your Unique Body (and Quiet That Critical Voice!)*. Carlsbad, CA: Gurze Books, p.114.

7 Use this link to get automatic results from the Compulsive Exercise Test (CET): www.jennischaefer.com/cet.

8 Darpinian, S. (2020, August 7) Disrupting Habits that Don't Help. Therapy Rocks! Episode 5. Accessed on 8/9/2021 at https://audioboom.com/posts/7651840-disrupting-habits-that-don-t-help.

9 Glasofe, D.R. and Steinglass, J. (2016, September 1) Disrupting the habits of anorexia: How a patient learned to escape the rigid routines of an eating disorder. *Scientific American*. Accessed on 8/9/2021 at www.scientificamerican.com/article/disrupting-the-habits-of-anorexia.

10 Darpinian, S. (2020, April 23) The Expert Clothes Encounter. Therapy Rocks! Episode 1. Accessed on 8/9/2021 at https://audioboom.com/posts/7564811-the-expert-clothes-encounter.

11 Chastain, R. (2017, June 13) Ragen Chastain and Exercise for All Bodies. Dietitians Unplugged Podcast, Episode 25. Accessed on 8/9/2021 at https://dietitiansunplugged.libsyn.com/episode-25-ragen-chastain-exercise-for-all-bodies.

12 Centers for Disease Control and Prevention (2020) Disability and Health Overview. Accessed on 8/9/2021 at www.cdc.gov/ncbddd/disabilityandhealth/disability.html.

13 Graham, N., Schultz, L., Mitra, S., and Mont, D. (2017) Disability in Middle Childhood and Adolescence. In: D.A.P. Bundy, N. de Silva, S. Horton, G.C. Patton, *et al.* (eds) *Child and Adolescent Health and Development*. 3rd edition. Washington, DC: The International Bank for Reconstruction and Development/The World Bank.

14 Mizunoya, S., Mitra, S., and Yamasaki, I. (2016) *Towards Inclusive Education: The Impact of Disability on School Attendance in Developing Countries*. Innocenti Working Paper No. 2016-03. Florence: UNICEF Office of Research.

Chapter 5

1   Mensinger, J.L., Calogero, R.M., Stranges, S., and Tylka, T.L. (2016) A weight-neutral versus weight-loss approach for health promotion in women with high BMI: A randomized-controlled trial. *Appetite 105*, 364–374. doi:10.1016/j.appet.2016.06.006.

2   Tylka, T. and Diest, A. (2013) The Intuitive Eating Scale-2: Item refinement and psychometric evaluation with college women and men. *Journal of Counseling Psychology 60*, 1, 137–153. doi:10.1037/a0030893.

3   Khasteganan, N., Lycett, D., Furze, G., and Turner, A.P. (2019) Health, not weight loss, focused programmes versus conventional weight loss programmes for cardiovascular risk factors: A systematic review and meta-analysis. *Systematic Reviews 8*, 1, 200. doi:10.1186/s13643-019-1083-8.

4   www.ellynsatterinstitute.org.

5   Darpinian, S. (2020, December 16) Diet-free Parenting. Therapy Rocks! Episode 10. Accessed on 8/9/2021 at https://audioboom.com/posts/7752627-diet-free-parenting.

6   Your Fat Friend (2020) We Have to Stop Thinking of Being "Healthy" as Being Morally Better. Accessed on 8/9/2021 at www.self.com/story/healthism.

7   Tresley, J. and Sheean P. (2008) Refeeding syndrome: Recognition is the key to prevention and management. *Journal of the Academy of Nutrition and Dietetics 108*, 12, 2105–2108. doi:10.1016/j.jada.2008.09.01516.

8   Rapaport, L. (2018) Dieting pressure in teen years tied to food and weight problems later. Reuters, March 6. Accessed on 8/9/2021 at www.reuters.com/article/us-health-teens-parents-dieting-idUSKCN1Gl2OC.

9   Fisher, J.O. and Birch, L.L. (1999) Restricting access to foods and children's eating. *Appetite 32*, 3, 405–419. doi:0.1006/appe.1999.0231.

10 Birch, L.L., Fisher, J.O., and Davison, K.K. (2003) Learning to overeat: Maternal use of restrictive feeding practices promotes girls' eating in the absence of hunger. *American Journal of Clinical Nutrition 78*, 2, 215–220. doi:10.1093/ajcn/78.2.215.

11 Musher-Eizenman, D.R., Holub, S.C., Hauser, J.C., and Young, K.M. (2007) The relationship between parents' anti-fat attitudes and restrictive feeding. *Obesity 15*, 8, 2095–2102. doi:10.1038/oby.2007.249.

12 Galmiche, M., Déchelotte, P., Lambert, G. and Tavolacci, M.P. (2019) Prevalence of eating disorders over the 2006–2018 period: A systematic literature review. *American Journal of Clinical Nutrition 109*, 5, 1402–1413. doi:10.1093/ajcn/nqy342.

13 Darpinian, S. (2020, December 16) Diet-free Parenting. Therapy Rocks! Episode 10. Accessed on 8/9/2021 at https://audioboom.com/posts/7752627-diet-free-parenting.

Chapter 7

1   Elgar, F.J., Craig, W., and Trites, S.J. (2013) Family dinners, communication, and mental health in Canadian adolescents. *Journal of Adolescent Health 52*, 4, 433–438. doi:10.1016/j.jadohealth.2012.07.012.

2   Miller, D.P., Waldfogel, J., and Han, W.J. (2012) Family meals and child academic and behavioral outcomes. *Child Development 83*, 6, 2104–2120. doi:10.1111/j.1467-8624.2012.01825.

3   Harrison, M.E., Norris, M.L., Obeid, N., Fu, M., Weinstangel, H., and Sampson, M. (2015) Systematic review of the effects of family meal frequency on psychosocial outcomes in youth. *Canadian Family Physician/ Medecin de famille canadien 61*, 2, e96–e106.

4   The Family Dinner Project: https://thefamilydinnerproject.org/fun/?_sft_post_tag=dinner-games-2.

5   Ding, L., Hamid, N., Shepherd, D., and Kantono, K. (2019) How is satiety affected when consuming food while working on a computer? *Nutrients 11*, 7, 1545. doi:10.3390/nu11071545.

6   Benetou, V., Kanellopoulou, A., Kanavou, E., Fotiou, A., *et al.* (2020) Diet-Related behaviors and diet quality among school-aged adolescents living in Greece. *Nutrients 12*, 12, 3804. doi:10.3390/nu12123804.

7   Przybylski, A.K. and Weinstein, N. (2013) Can you connect with me now? How the presence of mobile communication technology influences face-to-face conversation quality. *Journal of Social and Personal Relationships 30*, 3, 237–246. 10.1177/0265407512453827.

8   NSF (n.d.) About NSF. Accessed on 8/9/2021 at www.nsf.org/consumer-resources/what-is-nsf-certification.

9   USP (n.d.) USP Verified Mark. Accessed on 8/9/2021 at www.usp.org/verification-services/verified-mark.

10 Informed Choice (n.d.) About Informed Choice. Accessed on 8/9/2021 at https://choice.wetestyoutrust.com/about-informed-choice.

11 Institute of Medicine, Food and Nutrition Board (2010) *Dietary Reference Intakes for Calcium and Vitamin D*. Washington, DC: National Academy Press.

12 Norman, A.W. and Henry, H.H. (2012) Vitamin D. In J.W. Erdman, I.A. Macdonald, and S.H. Zeisel (eds) *Present Knowledge in Nutrition*, 10th edn. Washington, DC: Wiley-Blackwell.

13 Jones, G. (2014) Vitamin D. In A.C. Ross, B. Caballero, R.J. Cousins, K.L. Tucker, and T.R. Ziegler (eds) *Modern Nutrition in Health and Disease*, 11th edn. Philadelphia, PA: Lippincott Williams & Wilkins.

14 Hancocks, N. (2020) Clear link between vitamin D deficiency and severity of coronavirus, say researchers. Nutra Ingredients. Accessed on 8/9/2021 at www.nutraingredients.com/Article/2020/04/28/Clear-link-between-vitamin-D-deficiency-and-severity-of-coronavirus-say-researchers.

15 Radujkovic, A., Hippchen, T., Tiwari-Heckler, S., Dreher, S., Boxberger, M., and Merle, U. (2020) Vitamin D deficiency and outcome of COVID-19 patients. *Nutrients 12*, 9, 2757. doi:10.3390/nu12092757.

16 Zemb, P., Bergman, P., Camargo, C.A. Jr, Cavalier, E., *et al.* (2020) Vitamin D deficiency and the COVID-19 pandemic. *Journal of Global Antimicrobial Resistance 22*, 133–134. doi:10.1016/j.jgar.2020.05.006.

Chapter 8

1   Neumark-Sztainer, D., Story, M., Perry, C., and Casey, M.A. (1999) Factors influencing food choices of adolescents: Findings from focus-group discussions with adolescents. *Journal of the American Dietetic Association* 99, 8, 929–937. doi:10.1016/S0002-8223(99)00222-9.

2   Ellyn Satter Institute (n.d.) Child feeding ages and stages. Accessed on 8/9/2021 at www.ellynsatterinstitute.org/how-to-feed/child-feeding-ages-and-stages.

3   Rampersaud, G.C., Pereira, M.A., Girard, B.L., Adams, J., and Metzl, J.D. (2005) Breakfast habits, nutritional status, body weight, and academic performance in children and adolescents. *Journal of the American Dietetic Association 105*, 5, 743–760 (quiz, pp.761–762). doi:10.1016/j.jada.2005.02.007.

Chapter 9

1   Darpinian, S. (2020, September 8) The Benefits of Boundaries. Therapy Rocks! Episode 6. Accessed on 8/9/2021 at https://audioboom.com/posts/7677693-the-benefits-of-boundaries.

2   Harris, R. (2014) The Complete Set of Client Handouts and Worksheets from ACT books by Russ Harris. Accessed on 8/9/2021 at https://thehappinesstrap.com/upimages/Complete_Worksheets_2014.pdf.

3   Adapted from Russ Harris Values Worksheet. Harris, R. (2008) Values Worksheet. Accessed on 8/9/2021 at https://thehappinesstrap.com/upimages/Values_Questionnaire.pdf.

4   Out of the FOG (n.d.) What to Do: A Toolbox of Ideas That Have Worked—Boundaries. Accessed on 8/9/2021 at https://outofthefog.website/what-to-do-2/2015/12/3/boundaries.

5   Schaeffer, B. (2009) *Is it Love or Is it Addiction?* Center City, MN: Hazelden, pp.43–56.

6   Levine, P.A. with Frederick, A. (1997) *Waking the Tiger: Healing Trauma.* Berkeley, CA: North Atlantic Books, p.19.

7   Schaeffer, B. (2009) *Is it Love or Is it Addiction?* Center City, MN: Hazelden.

Chapter 10

1   Gilliam, S. and Pipher, P.D.M. (2019) *Reviving Ophelia 25th Anniversary Edition: Saving the Selves of Adolescent Girls.* New York, NY: Riverhead Books.

2   Coyne, S.M., Hurst, J.L., Dyer, W.J., Hunt, Q., *et al.* (2021) Suicide risk in emerging adulthood: Associations with screen time over 10 years. *Journal of Youth and Adolescence.* doi:10.1007/s10964-020-01389-6.

3   Makwana, B., Lee, Y., Parkin, S., and Farmer, L. (2018) Self-esteem: The relationship between body dissatisfaction and social media in adolescent and young women. *The Inquisitive Mind*, 35. Accessed on

8/9/2021 at www.in-mind.org/article/selfie-esteem-the-relationship-between-body-dissatisfaction-and-social-media-in-adolescent.

4   Rideout, V., Fox, S., Peebles, A., and Robb, M.B. (2021) *Coping with COVID-19: How Young People Use Digital Media to Manage Their Mental Health*. San Francisco, CA: Common Sense and HopeLab. Accessed on 8/9/2021 at www.commonsensemedia.org/sites/default/files/uploads/research/2021-coping-with-covid19-full-report.pdf.

5   Markey, C. (2020) Build body confidence while using social media. *Psychology Today*. Accessed on 8/9/2021 at www.psychologytoday.com/intl/blog/smart-people-don-t-diet/202005/build-body-confidence-while-using-social-media.

6   Rounds, E.G. and Stutts, L.A. (2020) The impact of fitspiration content on body satisfaction and negative mood: An experimental study. *Psychology of Popular Media 10*, 2, 267–274. doi:10.1037/ppm0000288.

7   Murray, S.B., Nagata, J.M., Griffiths, S., Calzo, J.P., *et al.* (2107) The enigma of male eating disorders: A critical review and synthesis. *Clinical Psychology Review 57*, 1–11. doi:10.1016/j.cpr.2017.08.001.

8   Herbozo, S., Tantleff-Dunn, S., Gokee-Larose, J., and Thompson, J.K. (2004) Beauty and thinness messages in children's media: A content analysis. *Eating Disorders 12*, 1, 21–34. doi:10.1080/10640260490267742.

9   Blond, A. (2008) Impacts of exposure to images of ideal bodies on male body dissatisfaction: A review. *Body Image 5*, 3, 244–250. doi:10.1016/j.bodyim.2008.02.003.

10 CNN (2021) Study: Girls who play with ultrathin dolls more likely to have body image issues. NBC. Accessed on 8/9/2021 at https://nbc-2.com/news/2021/03/11/study-girls-who-play-with-ultrathin-dolls-more-likely-to-have-body-image-issues.

11 www.nationaleatingdisorders.org.

12 Bench, S.W. and Lench, H.C. (2013) On the function of boredom. *Behavioral Sciences 3*, 3, 459–472. doi:10.3390/bs3030459.

13 Park, G., Lim, B.C., and Oh, H.S. (2019) Why being bored might not be a bad thing after all. *Academy of Management Discoveries 5*, 1, 78–92. doi:10.5465/amd.2017.0033.

14 Kuzma, C. (2020) What is healthy body image, anyways? *Women's Running*. Accessed on 8/9/2021 at www.womensrunning.com/health/wellness/healthy-body-image-defined.

15 Darpinian, S. (2020, May 21) Are The Kids Alright? Therapy Rocks! Episode 2. Accessed on 8/9/2021 at https://audioboom.com/posts/7588525-are-the-kids-alright.

Chapter 11

1   Almeida, L. (2020) Reduce body checking with 2 easy steps. Verywell Mind. Accessed on 8/9/2021 at www.verywellmind.com/reduce-body-checking-with-two-easy-steps-1138366.

2   Verplanken, B. and Orbell, S. (2003) Reflections on past behavior: A self-report index of habit strength. *Journal of Applied Social Psychology 33*, 6, 1313–1330. doi: 10.1111/j.1559-1816.2003.tb01951.x.
3   Tomasulo, D. (2020) *Learned Hopefulness: The Power of Positivity to Overcome Depression*. Oakland, CA: New Harbinger Publications, p.11.
4   Darpinian, S. (2021, February 2) Why Hope Is So Important in 2021. Therapy Rocks! Episode 12. Accessed on 8/9/2021 at https://audioboom.com/posts/7788973-why-hope-is-so-important-in-2021.
5   Darpinian, S. (2021, July 28) Personal communication.

Conclusion

1   Darpinian, S., Sterling, W., and Aggarwal, S. (2018) *No Weigh! A Teen's Guide to Positive Body Image, Food, and Emotional Wisdom*. London: Jessica Kingsley Publishers, p.185.

Index

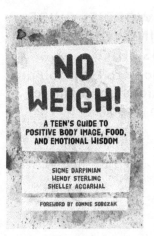

NO WEIGH!
A Teen's Guide to Positive Body Image, Food, and Emotional Wisdom

Signe Darpinian, Wendy Sterling, and Shelley Aggarwal

Foreword by Connie Sobczak

£14.99 | $20.95 | 192PP | PB | ISBN 978 1 78592 825 3 | eISBN 978 1 78450 946 0

This workbook has everything you need to achieve connected eating, body positivity and balanced exercise. It will help you stay well informed about how bodies change emotionally and physically in the teen years, and why good nutrition is critical for growth and development. It debunks any myths about diets and "forbidden" foods and also gives you the tools and strategies to avoid potential triggers of disordered eating.

No Weigh! A Teen's Guide to Positive Body Image, Food, and Emotional Wisdom will help you develop a lifelong healthy relationship with your food! We eat every day, so why not eat with pleasure, joy and happiness?

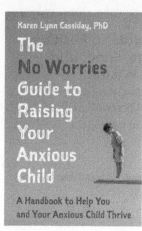

THE NO WORRIES GUIDE TO RAISING YOUR ANXIOUS CHILD
A Handbook to Help You and Your Anxious Child Thrive
Karen Lynn Cassiday, PhD

£12.99 | $18.95 | 208PP | PB | ISBN 978 1 78775 887 2 | eISBN 978 1 78775 888 9

This two-in-one handbook will help you to understand your child's anxiety and how to ease it, while also showing you how to reconcile your own fears and worries that come with raising an anxious child.

Tips and strategies from evidence-based therapies, such as CBT, ACT and exposure therapy, are paired in this guide with humorous, thoughtful and honest anecdotes of the author's own life and parenting experiences. Challenging modern cultural pressures to be a "perfect parent" and warning against the trap of over-accommodation, Dr Cassiday gives advice on how to embrace imperfection and uncertainty and to build resilience, compassion and gratitude so that anxiety can take the back seat in your family.

With a focus on acceptance and growth rather than "curing," this book will help you and your child to thrive and find joy even during the worst bouts of anxiety.

Karen Lynn Cassiday, PhD, ACT, is a clinical psychologist and Managing Director of The Anxiety Treatment Center of Greater Chicago. She is also Past President of The Anxiety and Depression Association of America (2016–2018) and is a Founding Fellow of the Academy of Cognitive Therapy (A-CBT).

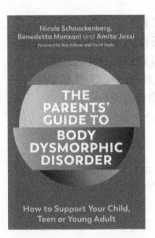

THE PARENTS' GUIDE TO BODY DYSMORPHIC DISORDER
How to Support Your Child, Teen or Young Adult

Nicole Schnackenberg, Benedetta Monzani and Amita Jassi

Foreword by Rob Wilson
and David Veale

£14.99 | $19.95 | 240PP | PB | ISBN 978 1 78775 113 2
| eISBN 978 1 78775 114 9

The first book offering support for parents and carers of children and young people with Body Dysmorphic Disorder (BDD), this guidebook explains the condition as well as the impact that it may have in education settings, family life and socialisation.

The guide begins by explaining how and why BDD emerges, before moving onto an exploration of how the mental health condition presents itself emotionally, psychologically, physically and behaviourally. It then offers practical advice and guidance for parents and carers on talking to their child about BDD, seeking professional treatment, considering medication, managing social media use, working with schools to build a recovery team and more.

The Parents' Guide to Body Dysmorphic Disorder is an essential guidebook for parents of children of children and young people with BDD.

Dr Nicole Schnackenberg is a Child, Community and Educational Psychologist and a trustee of the BDD Foundation. Nicole lives in Leigh-on-Sea, UK.

Dr Amita Jassi is a Consultant Clinical Psychologist at the National and Specialist OCD, BDD and Related Disorder Service for Children and Young People (South London and Maudsley NHS Trust). She lives in London, UK.

Dr Benedetta Monzani is a clinical psychologist at the National and Specialist OCD, BDD and Related Disorder Service for Children and Young People (South London and Maudsley NHS Trust). She lives in London, UK.

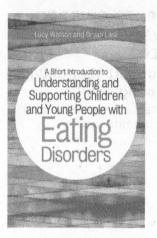

A SHORT INTRODUCTION TO UNDERSTANDING AND SUPPORTING CHILDREN AND YOUNG PEOPLE WITH EATING DISORDERS

Lucy Watson and Bryan Lask

£13.99 | $19.95 | 112PP | PB | ISBN 978 1 84905 627 4 | eISBN 978 1 78450 102 0

Increasing numbers of children and young people are presenting for treatment of an eating disorder, but there are many different types and they are often confused, making it difficult to know what support to offer.

This easy-to-read guide presents all the vital information on a range of eating disorders: anorexia nervosa, bulimia nervosa, selective eating, and avoidant and restrictive intake disorders. Each eating disorder is clearly defined, making it easy to draw distinctions between them. The book covers their origins, characteristics and typical development, letting teachers and parents know what signs to look out for. There is practical advice on how to help young people, strategies for overcoming common difficulties, as well as information on available treatments. Vignettes feature throughout to help teachers and parents apply knowledge to real-life situations.

This is an essential resource for teachers and parents of children and young people with eating disorders.

Lucy Watson is an Assistant Psychologist at the Michael Rutter Centre, Maudsley Hospital. She is the Editorial Assistant for the journal *Advances in Eating Disorders: Theory, Research & Practice*.

Professor Bryan Lask was Emeritus Professor of Child and Adolescent Psychiatry at St George's, University of London, UK, Medical Director at Rhodes Farm, Care UK, and Honorary Consultant Psychiatrist at Great Ormond Street Hospital for Children.